tao

long life

tao paths

long life

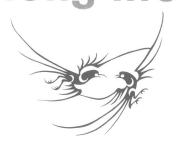

**Andrews McMeel
Publishing**

Kansas City

Contents

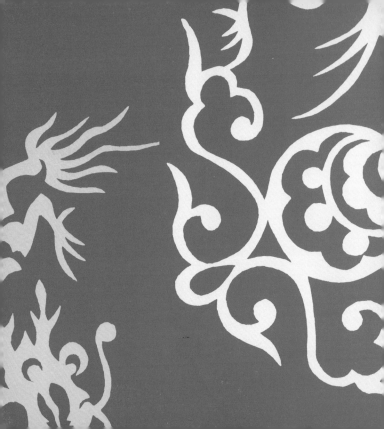

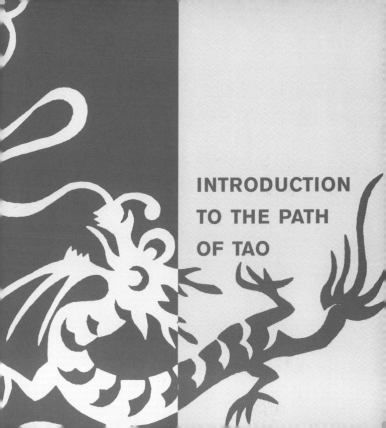

INTRODUCTION TO THE PATH OF TAO

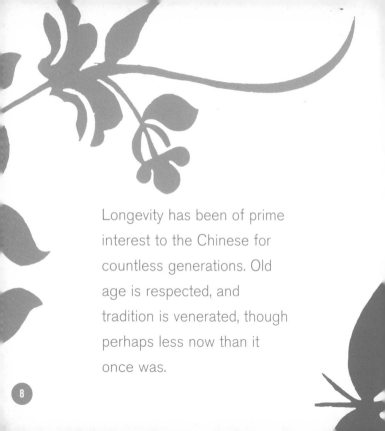

Longevity has been of prime interest to the Chinese for countless generations. Old age is respected, and tradition is venerated, though perhaps less now than it once was.

But the quest for long life is still very much in the forefront of the minds of modern Chinese as well as for everyone else.

To live long and prosper is the hope of everyone, regardless of nationality or race.

But while technological advances of the modern age have enhanced the life expectancy for most of us at the same time, the ills and complaints of living in this modern age have made life extremely challenging.

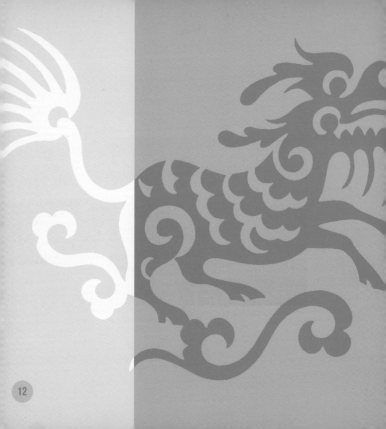

The Path of Tao is one of wholeness, balance, and harmony. It began eight thousand years ago in China, yet continues today wherever anyone follows these basic principles. It is less a religion and more a philosophy. It is a way to work *with* change rather than against it.

The Path of Tao is the Path of least resistance, of going with the flow of Nature (*wu wei*). It uses the metaphor of water, which adapts itself to the shape of whatever container it finds

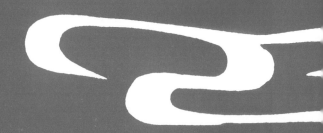

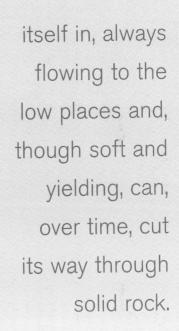

itself in, always
flowing to the
low places and,
though soft and
yielding, can,
over time, cut
its way through
solid rock.

Lao Tzu, the great ancient sage of Tao, said that the Path of Tao is one of seeing simplicity in the complicated and achieving greatness in small things. It is a Path that respects and even honors the Value of Worthlessness and the Wisdom of Foolishness.

Chuang Tzu, great sage of Tao, says, "Those who follow the Tao are strong in body, clear of mind, and sharp of sight and hearing. They do not fill their mind with anxieties and are flexible in adjusting to external conditions."

The Path of Tao is a way of life followed by the peasant, the farmer, the gentleman philosopher, and the artist. It is a way of deep reflection and learning from Nature, which is considered the highest teacher.

The Path of Tao offers us a simple, practical way of being and living, a way of comporting ourselves on our journey between birth and death and beyond. In wonderfully illustrative texts such as the *Tao Te Ching* and *Chuang Tzu*, we can find inspiration, illumination, and expedient advice on life, death, and all that lies between.

In Chinese medicine practices, we can find cure and comfort for many modern and not-so-modern ills and complaints. The practices of *chi kung* and *tai chi* can give us ways to stabilize and balance our bodies, allowing us to lead long-lasting and healthy lives. Taoist advice on sexuality and relationships can guide us gracefully through the difficult labyrinth of human sexuality.

And through Taoist spiritual and meditation practices, we may finally arrive at that precious point of power described in the Taoist tradition as Returning to the One—the source of our own being as well as beingness itself.

The *Tao Paths* series offers quotes gleaned from the traditional Taoist works as well as jewels of wisdom from contemporary Taoist masters.

Alongside these words of wisdom you will find stories to delight, mystify, and enlighten you to the deep layers of Taoist thought and practice.

Tao Paths covers a wide range of Taoist tradition and explores the ways in which the ancient sages as well as the modern masters have given us tools and practices to plumb the depths of our being and reunite us with our eternal source, the Tao itself.

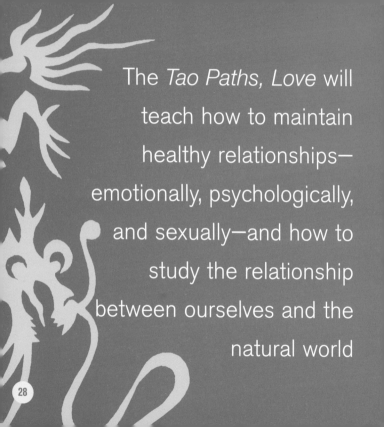

The *Tao Paths, Love* will teach how to maintain healthy relationships—emotionally, psychologically, and sexually—and how to study the relationship between ourselves and the natural world around us and the infinite depth of our own internal world.

Tao Paths, Harmony teaches how to be at one with the world around us.

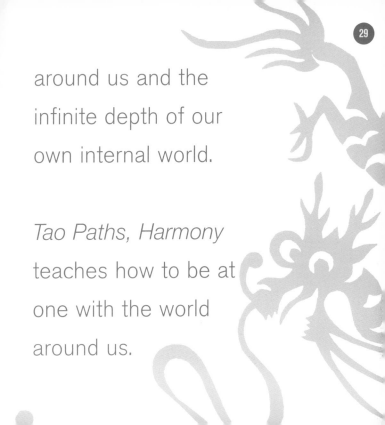

Tao Paths, Long Life teaches how to achieve a long and healthy life and how to live fully in each moment.

Tao Paths,
Good Fortune
explores the
realms of destiny,
karma, and good
fortune.

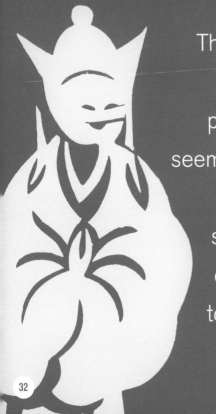

The problems of today are real, profound, often seem unresolvable, and call for something that can be applied to everyday life.

The Path of Tao
offers not a way out,
but a way through.
Its advice and
wisdom is real and
eminently applicable,
regardless of race,
religion, or gender.

What the ancient men and women of Tao learned through countless years of observation and practice can be just as useful today as it was in the time of the legendary Yellow Emperor.

Remember that the Path of Tao is not just an ancient, foreign, mystical path; it is a cross-cultural, nonsexist, practical, and even scientific way of viewing the world

and our place within it.
Its practices and philosophy
work on many different
levels—physical, emotional,
psychological, and spiritual.

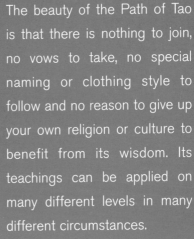

The beauty of the Path of Tao is that there is nothing to join, no vows to take, no special naming or clothing style to follow and no reason to give up your own religion or culture to benefit from its wisdom. Its teachings can be applied on many different levels in many different circumstances.

In China, there are temples of Taoism, a religious form of Tao (*tao jio*), complete with priests, liturgy, and rituals. But the original philosophical form of Taoism (*tao jia*) was intended as a way of life. It is this form of Taoism that we will be working with.

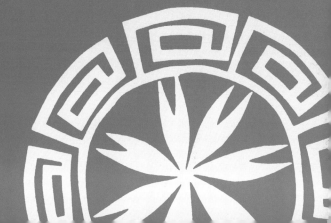

The roots of Tao go back thousands of years: the knowledge gleaned over the centuries can be as helpful for the modern world as in the Tang Dynasty. It can guide us onto the path of least resistance and help us find a way to work with the currents of change and renewal, and allow us to feel a sense of connection to the sacred.

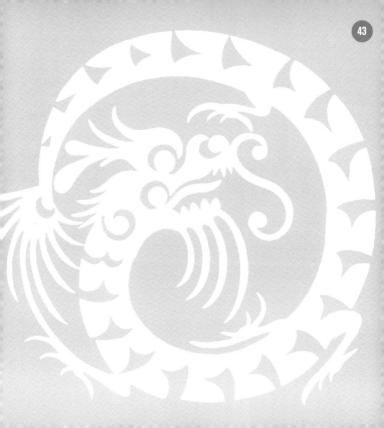

In *Tao Paths to Long Life* you will find inspiration and advice for contemplation and reflection, as well as practical instruction on using the traditional methods of Chinese medicine, working with diet and nutrition, working with energy or *chi*, balancing your emotions, and dealing with adversity when it arises.

This book will explore what
the Taoists have to say
about death and dying,
because no matter how long
a life we lead, we will all
have to face death one day.

You will meet many strange and wonderful characters in these pages—from the lofty wisdom of Lao Tzu to the often ridiculous metaphors of Chuang Tzu to the down-to-earth tales of Lieh Tzu.

In between, you will meet
hunchbacks, cripples, lords
and servants, wise sages, and
foolish seekers after Truth.

But pay attention, you may
meet yourself here.

**To hear of the Tao in the morning
is to die content at nightfall.**

CONFUCIUS

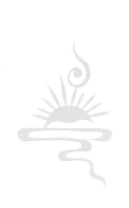

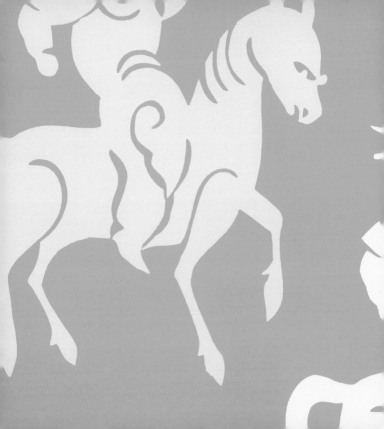

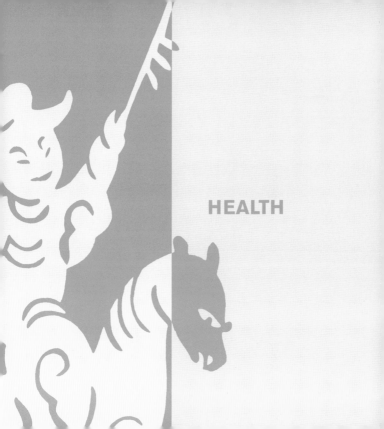

HEALTH

Chinese medicine has roots going back thousands of years, beginning with the ancient shaman healers of the Neolithic age. It has many variations and branches, including herbs, acupuncture, massage, bodywork, and *chi gong*. Practiced worldwide; it is used in clinics, hospitals, and people's homes.

It does not have all the answers, and modern Taoists advocate a combination of Western medicine and technology and the holistic approach of Chinese medicine—using each where it has its greatest application. In an emergency you don't want an acupuncturist! But afterward, acupuncture is a wonderful way to quicken the healing process and can be a great help with pain management.

Don't wish for perfect health. In perfect health there is greed and wanting. So an ancient said, "Make good medicine from the suffering of sickness."

Taoist medicine has its origin in the ancient Taoist philosophy, which views a person as an energy system wherein body and mind are unified, each influencing and balancing the other.

HUA CHING NI

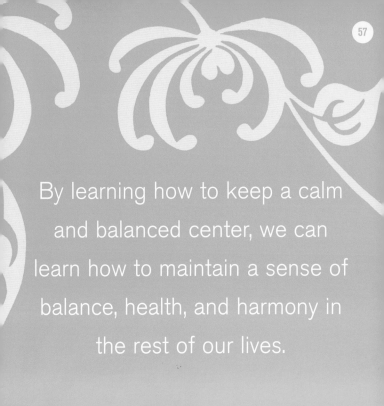

By learning how to keep a calm
and balanced center, we can
learn how to maintain a sense of
balance, health, and harmony in
the rest of our lives.

Taoists do not study disease;
they study life and health and
how to maintain them.

STEPHEN J. CHANG

The Taoist path to health and longevity is to keep a balance between yin and yang, and of the five elements or phases.

Regarding the human body as a machine made up of separate parts may work in a laboratory setting but when we are dealing with health issues it is important to view our body as a whole system, each part interdependent and interacting with the others.

The human system is a microcosm of nature and the cosmos; health and longevity can only be cultivated by harmonizing the human system with the rhythms of Heaven and Earth.

DANIEL REID

Yellow Emperor: I have heard that men of great antiquity lived over 200 years, and that men of middle antiquity lived up to 120 years. But today men often die before the age of 30. These days, so few men are relaxed and at ease with themselves, and so many suffer from diseases. What is the reason for this?

Plain Girl: The reason men die so young today is that they do not know the secrets of Tao.

CLASSIC OF THE PLAIN GIRL

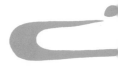

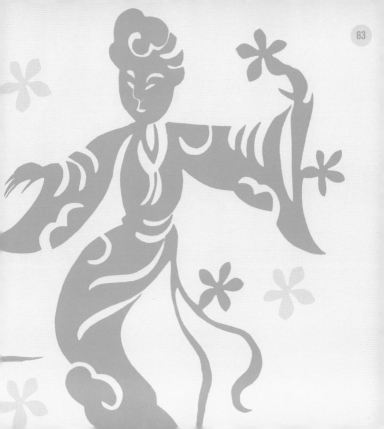

Indeed, the more "advanced" a society becomes, the shorter grow the lives of its members.

DANIEL REID

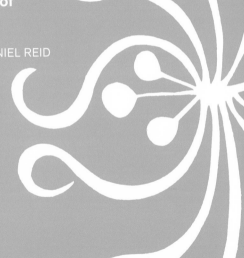

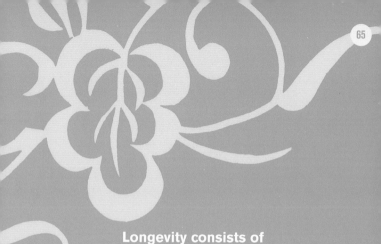

Longevity consists of maintaining one's health, slowing down the aging process, living without illness and pain, and dying peacefully without bothering other people.

HUAI CHIN NAN

Most people cram as many experiences and accomplishments as possible into one short life span. Taoists try to slow everything down, thereby extending their life.

When a man is young, he does not understand Tao. Even if he hears or reads about it, he is unlikely to fully believe or practice it. When he grows old and vulnerable, then he realizes the significance of Tao, but it is too late, because he is too sick to benefit from it.

SUN SSU-MO

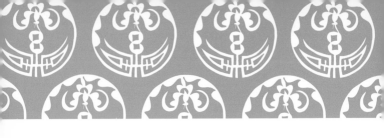

Don't wait until you're
unhealthy to become
concerned about your health.
Start when you are still healthy
and it will be so much easier
to maintain that good health.

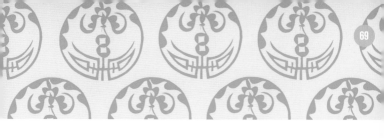

The Chinese method is thus holistic,
based on the idea that no single
part can be understood except in its
relation to the whole.

TED KAPTCHUCK

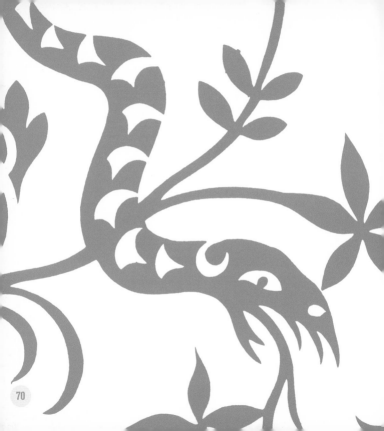

To be healthy is not simply
a matter of not being ill.
To be healthy is to be
balanced, grounded,
strong, and clear of mind.

**Medicine and sickness
mutually correspond. The
whole universe is medicine.
What is the self?**

YUN MEN

To know that one does not know is the highest wisdom.
Not to know that one does not know
Is a disease.
When one recognizes this as a disease
One can be free from disease.

LAO TZU

Why do some people
succumb to illness and
disease and not others;
why do we get sick on one
day and not another?

Disease occurs when one is inharmonious, either internally or externally. We are all exposed to disease every day.

The key to good health is moderation in all things, both physically and emotionally.

We get sick when we are moving too fast, when we are not paying attention, when we are ungrounded and unbalanced.

Avoid extreme emotion of all kinds, especially as you grow older. Nothing drains energy from the body as rapidly, nor disrupts the functional harmony of vital organs as completely, as strong outbursts of emotion.

LEE CHING YUEN

Nowadays everyone in the world is deluded about right and wrong and confused about benefit and harm; because so many people share this sickness, no one perceives that it is a sickness.

LIEH TZU

Sickness and health are not simply physical states that the methods of science will eventually analyze completely and make understandable. They are rooted in the deepest and most mysterious strata of Being.

ANDREW WEIL

We are all individuals. What may work for one person will not necessarily work for another. It is important to learn your own personal path to healing.

It is important to let go of any feelings of shame or guilt about being sick. Sometimes it is possible to trace the root of the sickness back to its source, sometimes it is not. In either case, remember that it is not your essential self that is sick, and do not view it as a punishment from on high.

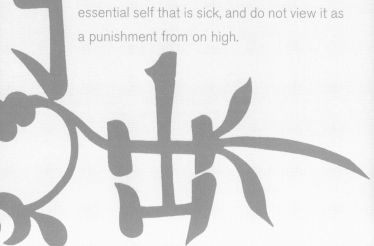

We need a system of medicine that considers the whole man and woman—their emotional and spiritual body as well as their physical body.

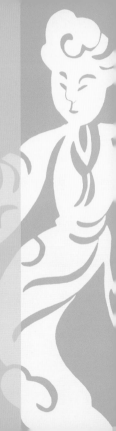

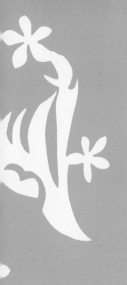

Modern man is solitary, and he is so of necessity and at all times, for every step toward a fuller consciousness of the present further removes him from his original participation with the mass of submersion in a common unconsciousness.

CARL JUNG

As we become ever more cut off from our roots and further removed from our sense of connection to the rest of the human race, our environment, and to the understanding of the interrelatedness of the universe itself, disease will become more and more prevalent.

You and I come forth as possibilities of essential nature, alone and independent as stars, yet reflecting and being reflected by all things.

ROSHI AIKTEN

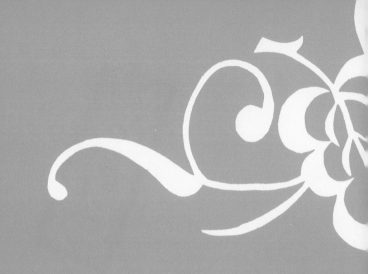

Health and well-being can be achieved only by remaining centered in spirit, guarding against the squandering of energy, promoting the constant flow of *qi* and blood, maintaining harmonious balance of yin and yang, adapting to the changing seasonal and yearly macrocosmic influences, and nourishing one's self preventively. This is the way to a long and happy life.

HUA CHING NI

Close your mouth.

Quiet your desires.

And your life will be full and healthy.

Keep talking

And meddling in the affairs of the world

And your life will be beyond hope.

LAO TZU

Taoists advocate taking it easy. Worrying about problems will not make them go away. Pushing too hard, stressing too much, even working too hard, can all bring negative results.

The physician must cure the disease the way it wants to be cured, not in the way he wants to cure it.

PARACELSUS

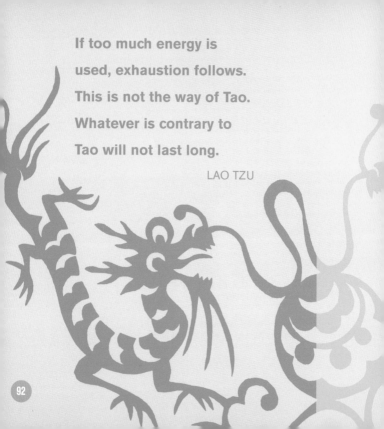

If too much energy is
used, exhaustion follows.
This is not the way of Tao.
Whatever is contrary to
Tao will not last long.

LAO TZU

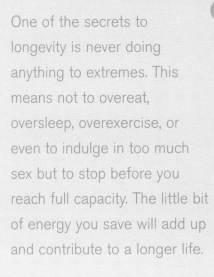

One of the secrets to longevity is never doing anything to extremes. This means not to overeat, oversleep, overexercise, or even to indulge in too much sex but to stop before you reach full capacity. The little bit of energy you save will add up and contribute to a longer life.

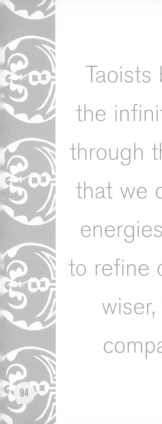

Taoists believe in reaching the infinite or enlightenment through the body. This means that we can use the intrinsic energies of our own bodies to refine ourselves to become wiser, lighter, and more compassionate beings.

By remaining calm and positive, we can affect our energy and thereby our health. It sounds simple but can be extremely challenging when we get sick.

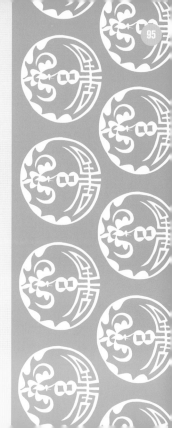

Disease can begin in many different ways. It can have an emotional basis, an energetic basis, a constitutional basis, an environmental basis, and even a spiritual basis. Follow the fruit back to its seed and deal with it there.

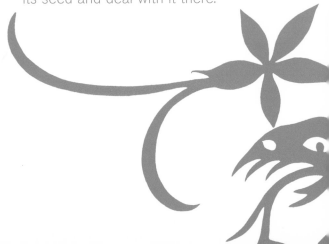

Chinese enlightenment is based on the idea that no single part can be understood except in its relation to the whole. A symptom, therefore, is not traced back to a cause, but is looked on as part of a totality.

By careful observation of
your daily cycles, you
can learn how to "read"
your energetic states
and tell what you need
for greater health.

If we pay attention
to our health when
it's good we will be
that much ahead
when something
does go wrong.

There is a growing interest today in the relationship of breathing to health and spiritual development. Unfortunately, few people who experiment with their breath understand the importance of "natural breathing."

MANTAK CHIA

The process of breathing, of the fundamental movement of inspiration and expiration, is one of the great miracles of existence. It not only unleashes the energies of life, but it also provides a healing pathway into the deepest recesses of our being.

DENNIS LEWIS

Natural breathing is when, as we inhale, our abdomen expands. Then, on exhalation, it contracts. This exercises the diaphragm and massages the internal organs, bringing *chi*, blood, and lymph to that area.

Most people breathe in a very shallow way, typically using only the top half of their lungs. Remember, the fight or flight state is one where our breathing becomes very shallow or even stops.

Many people breathe in a shallow way all the time, thereby keeping themselves in a chronic fight or flight state. By doing simple breathing exercises, we can change the way we breathe at all times, even when we're sleeping.

To breathe is to live. To inhale fully is to live fully, to manifest the full range and power of our inborn potential for vitality in everything that we sense, feel, think, and do.

DENNIS LEWIS

Sit on a cushion or chair and practice breathing as slowly and fully as you can. Imagine a ball of *chi* in your lower abdomen. Feel it expanding and contracting each time you inhale and exhale—energizing this area. The Taoists believe that one must build a strong foundation before attempting higher practices.

To inhale fully is to empty ourselves, to open ourselves to the unknown, to be expired. It is through a deepening awareness of the ever-changing rhythms of this primal process that we begin to awaken our inner healing powers—the energy of wholeness.

DENNIS LEWIS

Go slowly. The sage is one who never seems to be in a hurry about anything, yet gets everything done.

Always begin
at the beginning.
This means beginning with
who you are right now,
how you are right now, and
where you are right now.

You should bring yourself to yourself
by yourself and realize that you can
change everything in your life by
changing yourself.

HUA CHING NI

It is when we are trying hard to be strong that we are at our weakest. If we learn to relax and soften we can find our greatest strength.

The principle of Taoist medicine is like when the water boils, you do not stop the boiling water by blowing on it; you have to stop the fuel that powers the fire.

HUA CHING NI

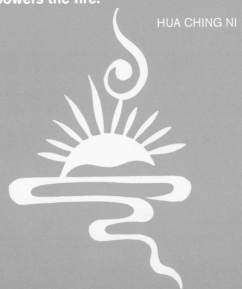

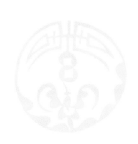

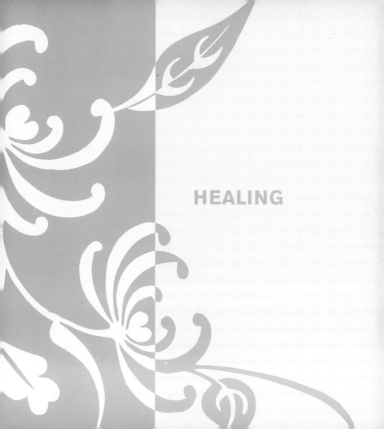

HEALING

Chinese medicine is based on the premise that everything is part of a web of infinite dimension, which connects everything in the universe. As part of this, we humans are influenced by everything that exists in the web: the stars, the weather, the food we eat, the sounds we hear, and all the things that touch us, including other humans. When we are in balance with these things and, most importantly, within ourselves, we are healthy. But we are seldom in perfect balance, even with our immediate surroundings, much less within ourselves.

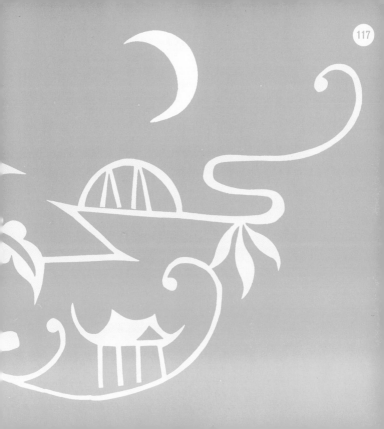

To gain balance and maintain it, the ancient Taoists have developed various treatments and practices. After all, the basis of a long life is to be healthy, happy, and whole!

To cure an illness that has already manifested itself is like starting to dig a well after one is already thirsty, or forging one's weapons after the battle has already begun.

NEIJING

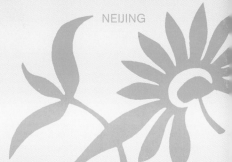

In China in previous times, a doctor would prescribe herbs and exercises to keep you healthy, and if you became sick and had to be treated, you did not pay. This was because, if the doctor was really doing his job, you would not need treatment.

Chinese medicine is concerned with changes
of state, dynamic and psychic factors,
function rather than substance.

MANFRED PORKERT

The true physician teaches the Tao—how to live. Traditional Chinese doctors are trained to cultivate well-being as well as to correct ill health. Planning ahead, Chinese medicine knows that storms interrupt clear weather and that illness stalks and gains a foothold when we are vulnerable. Its strategy is to enable us to withstand the storm without becoming disabled by it and to accumulate resources in times of good weather, peace, and plenty.

HARRIET BEINFIELD AND EFREM KORNGOLD

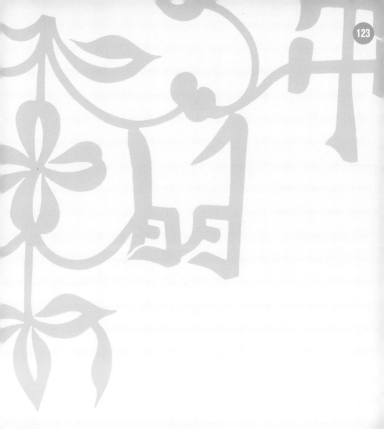

The great effectiveness of Chinese medicine is as a preventative. It is concerned with lifestyle and not just treatment. In this case, a proper balance of diet, sleep, sexual habits, environment, emotional state, and the ability to deal with stress are very important.

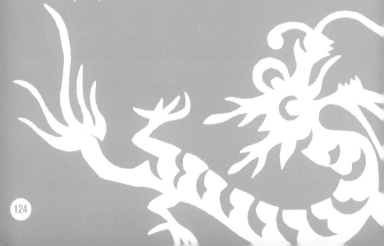

Lieh Tzu tells us about a gentleman of Yang Li who had lost his memory. He just sat in a chair without moving and hardly eating, did not know who he was, and did not recognize anyone around him. His family had called in all kinds of healers and diviners to cure him, all to no avail. Finally, when they had given up all hope, a Confucian scholar appeared, saying that if they would sign over half their property to him he would cure the old man.

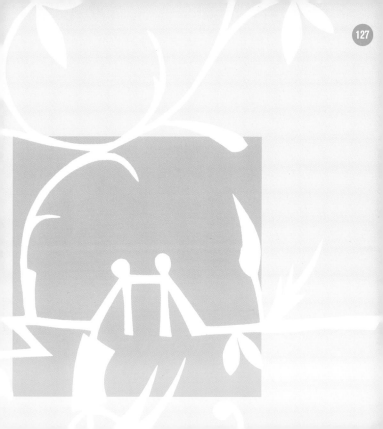

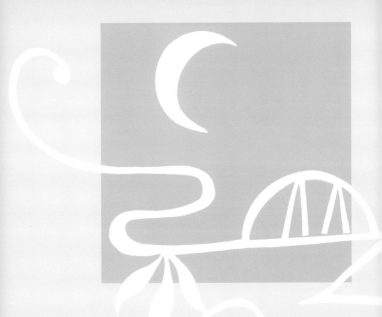

"This disease cannot be treated by the usual methods," he told them. "He must be cured by having his mind restored and his thoughts changed; then there is a chance that he can recover."

He proceeded to strip the old man and hide his clothing. The old man then began to look for them. Then the scholar began to starve him and he began to look for food. Finally he shut him up in the dark and the poor man began searching for light.

The scholar was delighted and told the man's family, "The sickness is curable. But my arts have been passed down secretly for generations and cannot be disclosed to outsiders. I must be alone with the patient for seven days."

And so the scholar and the patient were shut up in a room for seven days and, at the end of the long week, the patient was cured. The only problem was that the old man woke up very angry.

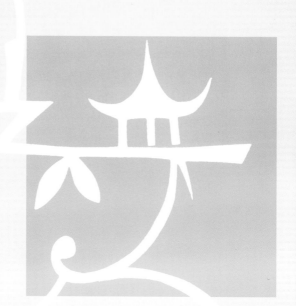

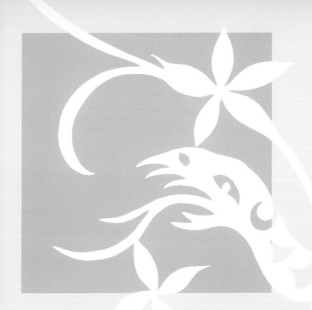

He dismissed his wife, beat up his sons, and chased the scholar away with a spear! After being arrested by the authorities and questioned about his strange behavior, he said, "When I lost my memory I was carefree and happy. I remembered nothing and so had no worries. I slept peacefully and didn't fret about anything. Now that I have recovered my memory of all my gains and losses, my fortunes and misfortunes, my joys and sorrows—all the myriad memories of a lifetime—I feel overwhelmed and dispirited. I was so much happier before I was cured!"

True healing occurs when we wake up from one kind of forgetfulness into another, when we can forget the limitations of the physical world and instead remember that we are, at all times, divine beings.

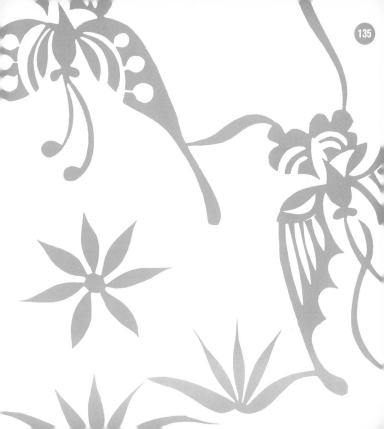

To the Taoists, the universe is divined into two polarities, yin and yang. In this way, all elements are paired and balanced with each other. These elements consist of primal qualities: male and female, night and day, sun and moon, moist and dry, dark and light. It is through the awareness and the experience of this interdependence and interrelationship that the universe, and we humans within it, remain in balance.

The attributes of yin are darkness, water, cold, rest, inward and downward direction, stillness, receptivity, and femaleness. The attributes of yang are brightness, heat, activity, upward and outward direction, aggressiveness, expansion, and maleness.

No one aspect is right for every situation; it is best to recognize and be willing to work with the ever-shifting balance of power in any situation. The secret is, as usual, to slow down, pay attention, and be true to your own nature or to the moment at hand.

We all have both yin and yang qualities within us. The balance between these two qualities is not static and concrete, but moving and shifting. At times our yin side asserts itself, at other times our yang does.

It is in keeping the proper balance of yin and yang influences and activities in our life that is the key to health and longevity.

Owing to the polarity of yin and yang, human energy, like all natural forces, is always moving, constantly transforming, ever active.

DANIEL REID

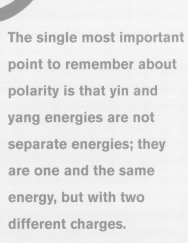

The single most important point to remember about polarity is that yin and yang energies are not separate energies; they are one and the same energy, but with two different charges.

MANTAK CHI

The principles of yin and yang suggests the inherent movement of the Tao. After all, life implies movement. In order to retain the flexibility that Lao Tzu talks about, we have to sustain the quality of movement in our lives.

By paying close attention to the qualities of yin and yang we can better determine when it is appropriate to act in a yang, or aggressive, manner and when it would be more appropriate to act in a yin, or reflective, manner.

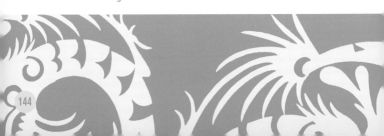

144

Some people have a predominantly yin nature and so would do better with yin type exercises such as walking, *tai chi*, and yoga. Others are of a more yang nature and find sports or running more natural.

Yin/Yang is the Way of heaven and earth, the fundamental principles of the myriad things, the father and mother of change and transformation, the root of conception and destruction.

SU-WEN

In the East, anyone can walk into a herbal pharmacy and purchase anything they require for either prevention or cure. Only when a patient fails to understand his own problem does he need to visit a doctor, who then prescribes therapy and advice that helps the patient cure himself. After all, no one is more familiar with your body than yourself.

DANIEL REID

What manifests is symptom.
What manifests as hidden is
well-being, that is, the well of
being from which the
symptom is born.

DIANNE M. CONNELLY

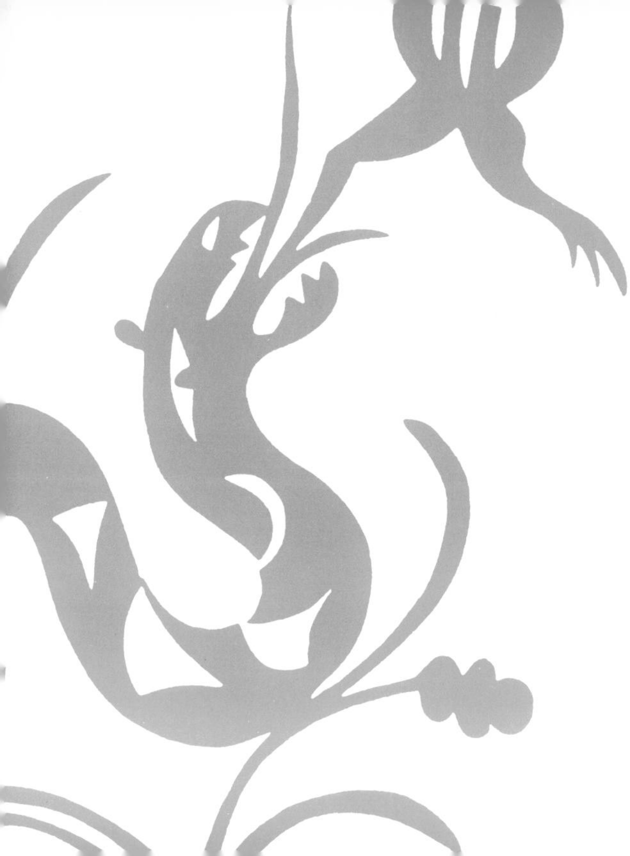

An important aspect of Taoist medicine is called the Five Element system, or more accurately, the Five Phases. This rather complicated system of correspondences should not be thought of in terms of absolute forms, but rather of processes of fire, earth, metal, water, and wood.

As in much of Taoist medicine and philosophy, these terms are relative and apt to shift in and out of each other, depending on their use.

According the Five Element system, all major organs are assigned to one of the specific elements, with a specific color, taste, emotion, season, etc. This system acknowledges that all parts of the body interact and are dependent on the others.

A weakness in one area will cause a corresponding weakness in another area. This means that in order to treat a disease it is important to be able to treat all the areas of disease.

A particular craving of a flavor or even a specific color can give an indication of the source of the disease or imbalance. At the same time, an overindulgence in one type of food or activity will also cause the whole system to become unbalanced, inviting disease.

**Taoists reason that
negative emotions can be
transformed to utilize
their lifeforce energy.**
MANTAK CHIA

The aim of Taoist medicine is to effect a balance, not only of yin and yang, but of all the phases of a human being, which include the physical, the emotional, the mental as well as the spiritual aspects of human life.

Keeping all these in perspective and in balance, we may live long and healthy lives.

The Five Elemental Energies (*wu hsing*), also translated as the Five Phases, are fundamental forces of nature created by the interplay of yin and yang on earth.

DANIEL REID

The liver corresponds to the color green—the green of new growth, of grasses, and of plants. It corresponds to the element of wood—the wood of plants and trees—and the season of spring. It is connected to the negative emotional state of anger and the positive emotional state of free flow and flexibility.

The heart corresponds to the color red, the element of fire, and the season of summer, when the fiery sun is at its highest aspect. The negative emotional aspect of the heart is hysteria while the positive is joy and creativity.

The spleen corresponds to the color yellow, the element earth, and the season of Indian summer or the time between seasons. It is where we feel our connection to the earth, or lack of it. The negative emotional state is worry or self-absorption and the positive emotional state is empathy and being grounded.

The lungs correspond to the color white, the element of metal or gold, and the season of autumn. The negative emotional state connected to the lungs is that of grief, while the positive emotional state is courage.

The kidneys correspond to the color blue-black, the element water, and the season of winter. The kidneys are also paired with the adrenal glands and are the repository of our *jing* or constitutional and sexual energy. The negative emotional state is fear, while the positive emotional state is that of willpower or backbone.

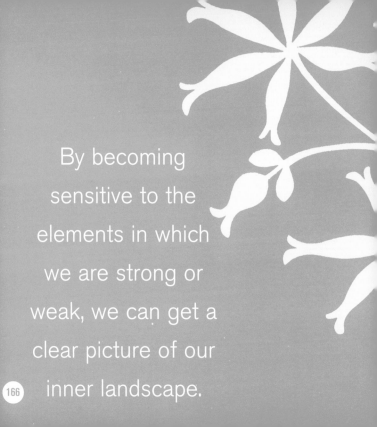

By becoming sensitive to the elements in which we are strong or weak, we can get a clear picture of our inner landscape.

A special attraction or repulsion of a certain flavor, season, or color can tell you a lot about your inbalances. Once you know that, you can take measures, using diet, herbs, energy practices, or even acupuncture.

Body, mind, and spirit are totally integrated in the Taoist view. Therefore, Chinese medicine finds that negative emotions, such as anger, fear, or cruelty, and excessive amounts of positive emotions, such as too much joy or excitement, can injure the organs and associated organs and cause disease.

MANTAK CHIA

All phenomena of
the world stimulate,
tone, subdue, or
depress one's
natural life force.

NEIJING

We can do energy practices, using the five elements system, to balance and tone our internal organs, and, through them, our emotions.

Sit or lie down quietly, breathing gently and slowly, from the belly, eyes closed.

Using your mind's eye, breathe the color green into your liver, located on your right side just under your rib cage. Smile down to your liver, acknowledging the wonderful job it does for you every day, filtering toxins from your body. See it as healthy and flexible. Instill in it the positive emotion of flexibility and kindness.

Breathe the color red into your heart. Again, smile down to it and fill it with love. Acknowledge it for the wonderful job it does, pumping blood throughout the circulation system of your body. See it as healthy and strong. Instill it with the positive emotions of joy and creativity.

Breathe the color white into your lungs. Smile down to them and feel them expanding and contracting, filled with good clean air and *chi*. Instill the positive emotions of courage and the ability to surrender deeply to life's challenges.

Breathe the color yellow into the spleen, located on the left side of your abdomen. This is where we feel our connection to the earth as well as to all other life-forms. Not only do we digest our food here but also our life experiences. Instill the positive emotions of empathy and compassion.

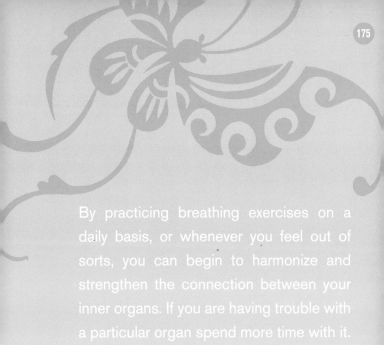

By practicing breathing exercises on a daily basis, or whenever you feel out of sorts, you can begin to harmonize and strengthen the connection between your inner organs. If you are having trouble with a particular organ spend more time with it. Just remember to always practice in a gentle manner.

From here we move to the kidneys, located in the lower back. Smile down to them and acknowledge them for their great work, along with the adrenal glands, in giving you your day-to-day energy as well as your sexual energy. Instill in them the positive qualities of gentleness and stability.

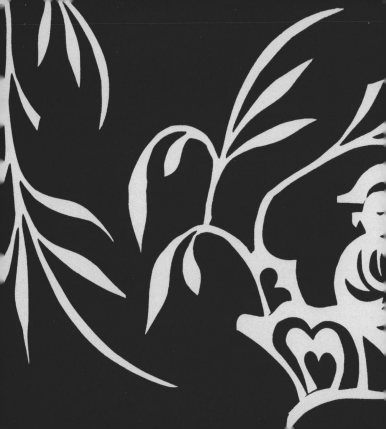

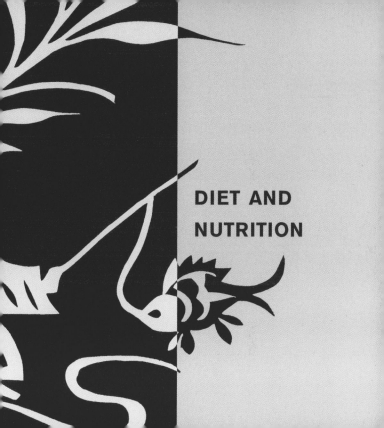

DIET AND NUTRITION

Diet and nutrition play a big part in longevity. If you want to live a long and healthy life, you need to take the proper nourishment. This can be a problem in Western society, with so much nutritionally empty "fast food" available.

The time that you save on eating these kinds of meals will only be lost to disease or a shortened life span. Instead, take the time to eat simple yet nourishing meals, full of whole grains and local produce. Also, never overeat. Keep yourself in the 70 to 80 percent full ratio. This way your stomach can more easily digest your meal.

There is no diet that is perfect for everyone. Some people do very well with a strict vegetarian or even vegan diet. Others may weaken and have their immune systems compromised by such a diet. They will need to add chicken or fish into their diet. Others do well with red meats.

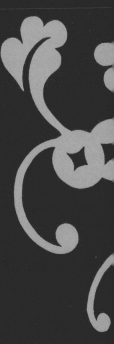

If you eat meat, it is important to seek out a source of organic or free-range meats. The amount of antibiotics and other dangerous additives found in commercial meats can be a serious health risk for those with a weak digestion or immune system.

We are all ultimately part of the food chain. To the Taoists, it is not considered more "spiritual" to be a vegetarian. In China today, there are some orders of religious Taoists who are vegetarians. But traditionally, all food is thought of as medicine.

Just as different people need different types of medicine, different body types need a different diet. By doing some research into your own body type and the general health of your digestive system you will be able to choose a diet that is ideal for you.

In traditional Chinese medicine, diet and nutrition remain important pillars of health and longevity and are regarded as crucial adjuncts to all branches of medical therapy.

DANIEL REID

Anyone, even a beggar,

is the same as an

Emperor during his meal.

The Master was traveling with some of her students. At one of their stops they were served the meat of a pig. The students were horrified to see the Master calmly eating this forbidden food. "Master," they cried, "is not the flesh of an animal forbidden by our order?"

The Master went on chewing slowly, clearly savoring the taste of the forbidden food. When she had finished she said, "Can you not see that to be given this delicacy was a great and honored gift from these poor people? No doubt it was given at great cost to them and with an attitude of humbleness and generosity. Who am I to spurn their gift? Besides," she said, taking another bite, "it is not what goes into your mouth that defiles you, but what comes out of it."

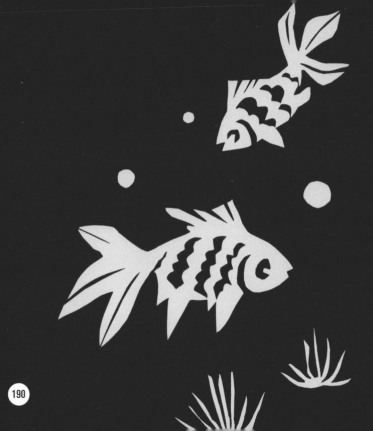

Do you know what kind of food is the most nourishing? The best nourishment comes from your relaxed, calm mind. If you eat food, but have a troubled mind, the results will not be good.

Remember the saying "You are what you eat"? By paying attention to what we eat we can affect both our health and our longevity. Diets high in refined flour, sugar, and caffeine will not lead to longevity.

By avoiding extreme temperatures in our food, neither too hot nor too cold, we can allow our digestive system to work more smoothly and efficiently. Basically, the digestive process is one of cooking. Because of this, it is plain to see that eating too many cold foods will slow down and hinder that process.

A truly good physician first finds out the cause of the illness, and having found that, he first tries to cure it by food. Only when food fails does he prescribe medication.

SUN SSU-MIAO

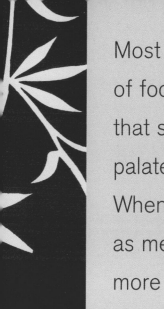

Most people only think of food as something that should please the palate or feed a craving. When we think of food as medicine we will be more careful of what we put into our bodies.

In Taoist medicine, foods are categorized according to the five elements; sweet (earth), bitter (fire), sour (wood), pungent (metal), and salty (water). It is said that each of the five organs (spleen, heart, liver, lungs, and kidneys) have an affinity for one of the five flavors.

In this way, specific flavors or foods can be used to balance, tone, and detoxify specific organs.

The best thing is to eat a little of everything and not a lot of anything.

HUA CHING NI

Assist your digestion by avoiding eating too much at one time or eating a heavy meal late in the day, and by not eating too many stimulating foods such as sugar and caffeine.

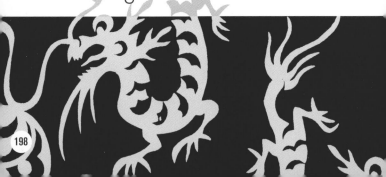

Exercising correctly can greatly help digestion and taking even a short walk after a meal will help.

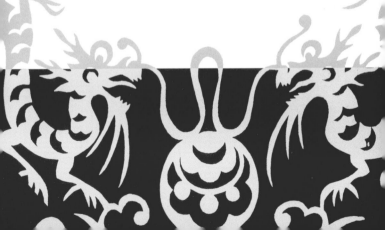

The simple exercises of *tai chi* and *chi gong* will keep your internal energies moving and help your body do its job in the best way possible.

To begin a healthier diet, change from drinking coffee to green tea. Green tea has less caffeine, none of the acids, and will give you a gentle lift without draining your adrenals. It has been found to lower cholesterol and reduce high blood pressure and the rate of lung cancer, even in smokers.

Tea is said to be a "Way" (Tao). This is because it is something one learns to appreciate through feeling, not though verbal instruction. If a person maintains a state of quietness, only then will he appreciate the quietness inherent in tea. If he is excited, he will never recognize the tea's quietness. For this reason it is said that "tea and meditation are one taste." If one's meditation is not single-pointed one will fail to appreciate the true qualities of tea.

POPCHONG SUNIM

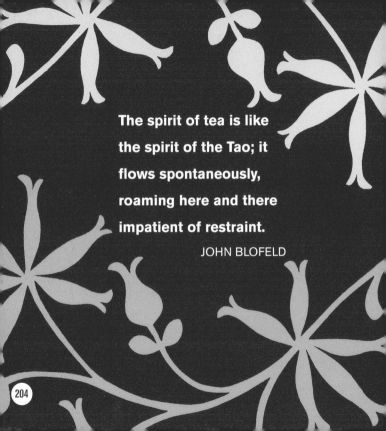

The spirit of tea is like
the spirit of the Tao; it
flows spontaneously,
roaming here and there
impatient of restraint.

JOHN BLOFELD

The Way of Tea, *Cha Tao*, is like much else on the Path of Tao. It involves quiet, introspection, an appreciation for the subtle and the simple, and the ability to surrender to the moment.

In ancient China, a whole philosophy called the Way of Tea was formed, in which tea masters were said to be able to not only correctly identify any tea and the region it came from, but were even able to tell which spring water was used!

Tea has some effect against cancer because it inhibits the formation or action of cancer-causing substances. Tea may block the action of nitrosamines which can cause cancer.

KIT CHOW AND IONE KRAMER

There is a famous story about Lu Yu, a famous tea master who was an expert on what kind of water was best for brewing tea. He actually wrote a book on twenty sources for the water to be used for brewing tea.

The best, he said, was from midstream on the Yangtze at Nanling. Once, on a trip on the river he was given water from that spot to taste. Upon tasting it Lu Yu said that the water was not from midstream but from closer to the shore.

"But that cannot be," said his host. "I am sure it was taken from midstream."

"Perhaps," conceded the master, "but there is some other kind of water mixed into it."

Later it was discovered that some of the water from the container had been lost when the boat had rocked and the servant had replaced it with some water taken from nearer the shore.

The first cup caresses my dry lips and throat,

The second shatters the walls of my

lonely sadness,

The third searches the dry rivulets of my

soul to find the stories of five thousand scrolls.

With the fourth the pain of past injustice

vanishes through my pores.

The fifth purifies my flesh and bone.

With the sixth I am in touch with the Immortals.

The seventh gives such pleasure I can hardly bear.

The fresh wind blows through my wings

As I make my way to Penglai. (Land of

the Immortals).

LU TONG

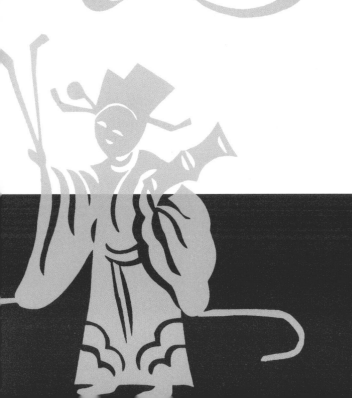

The Taoist sages were very adept at observing nature, and they learned the use of many herbs by watching what animals ate when they were injured or sick.

Over 5,000 years ago the great emperor Shen Nong discovered the properties of a great many herbs by ingesting them himself, a brave though potentially dangerous way of going about it!

Originally herbs were thought of as food—highly nutritious, beneficial food. The ancient Chinese formulas, or recipes, spoke of herbal "soups" rather than teas. Herbs were eaten as part of the daily meals, cooked into soups or broths, or eaten as salads.

There were, of course, purely medicinal herbs, but for the most part, herbs were used as a means of strengthening or maintaining the integrity of the body. The Chinese also use a great many substances in their pharmacopoeia, some which may be surprising to the Western reader.

A compendium by the famous physician Li Shi-zhen, published in 1596, includes 1,892 entries: 1,173 are botanical ingredients, 444 are zoological or animal derived, and 275 are derived from minerals. The most recently published pharmacopoeia lists 5,767 entries!

Over thousands of years of observation, exploration, and experimentation, the Chinese herbalists were able to find specific uses for an incredible range of substances, from the lovely chrysanthemum flower to the lowly earthworm.

Herbs give everlasting strength, whereas regular foods give only temporary strength.

STEPHEN T. CHANG

Chinese herbs are almost always used in combination with other herbs in very specific formulas, many of which are thousands of years old. It is in the way the herbs work synergistically with each other that gives the formula its efficacy.

Always consult a properly trained herbalist or Chinese physician before starting a Chinese herbal program.

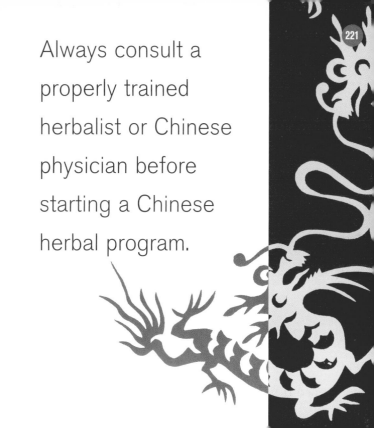

Herbs can be used for spiritual cultivation, called *lian dan shu* or the art of alchemy. The herbs are used to open spiritual centers in the body, removing negative or dark energies and dissolving emotional congestion.

Truth is simple; Nature is simple. It is not in strong colors or flavors or complicated structures, but in simplicity that the essence is attained through years of cultivation and development.

Then you are able to appreciate simplicity. This is the true Taoist art.

HUA CHING NI

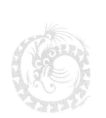

WORKING WITH ENERGY

Chi (sometimes spelled *qi*) can be thought of as the basic life force, energy, *prana*, breath, or simply vital energy. It is the very stuff of life. It is what animates us, what gives us life. It warms us, keeps our organs in their place, and directs all our movements.

Everything that is alive has *chi*—humans, animals, plants, trees, mountains, the very air that we breathe. Death is the point where the *chi* leaves the body. We can affect our *chi* by doing special energy practices like *chi gong* (sometimes spelled *qigong*). This is a practice to access, circulate, and then store *chi* in our body.

There are different kinds of *chi* with different jobs to do. For example, there is protective *chi* or *wei chi*. It lies like an invisible electric shield between the skin and the muscles. Its job is to keep out invading pathogens, or "outside evils." When our *wei chi* is low, our resistance to colds, flus, or more serious viral invasion is weakened.

Another kind of *chi* is meridian *chi*, which travels the pathways (called meridians or channels) throughout our bodies, linking organs to each other and to organ systems, and helping the blood flow and stay within its channels. Meridian *chi* is what acupuncturists tap into when they insert their needles.

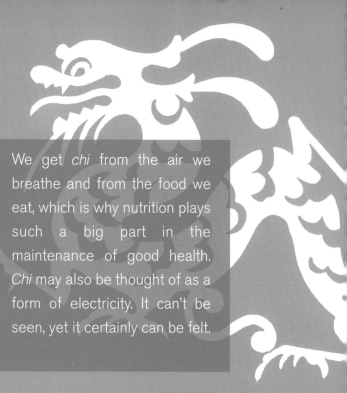

We get *chi* from the air we breathe and from the food we eat, which is why nutrition plays such a big part in the maintenance of good health. *Chi* may also be thought of as a form of electricity. It can't be seen, yet it certainly can be felt.

You can think of the meridian system in the human body as an electrical system complete with junctions, fuse boxes, and miles of wiring, all connecting into one great multilevel energy circuit.

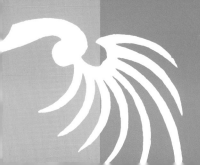

The term *chi gong* is made up of two characters. *Chi* meaning energy and *gong*, which means work or something that takes effort and time. Thus the term *chi gong* means working with your energy.

Chi gong is a series of movements, both internal and external, that directly activates or helps a smooth flow of *chi* or vital force throughout the body.

HUA CHING NI

Qigong began with the first breath of God. This inspiration, this first breath, is the first *Qigong*. It was the moment when nonbeing made the transition into being. This is the power of God. We use the character *wu* and *ji* to create the *Wuji*. It can refer to God; it can refer to "endlessness"; it can refer to the "end of nonbeing." It is all these things. This is the essence of *Qigong* . . . to bring you into the awareness of the infinite nature of your soul.

DUAN ZHI LIANG

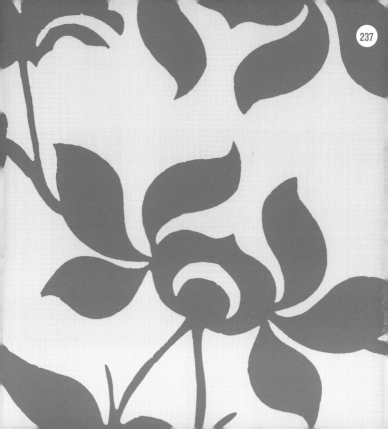

Your body, in cooperation with your mind and spirit, is marvelously blessed with miraculous and self-healing abilities. The body is the temple of your life. Mind and spirit are the dwellers within the temple. Mind and spirit maintain the temple.

Mind's intelligence and spirit's inspiration vitalize and quicken the body. The three together—body, mind, and spirit—cooperate to produce the most profound medicine ever known in the history of the human race, right within you.

ROGER JAHNKE

To achieve spiritual immortality, one must first take proper care of the body as a basic vehicle of practice.

DANIEL REID

There are many different types of *chi gong*, some quite vigorous, some sublimely simple. No matter your age, gender, or health situation, there is a practice that is just right for you.

It is very difficult, if not impossible, to do high spiritual practices if you are ill, depressed, or have no energy. The Taoists believe that one must build up the energy of the body first, then one will be able to do more rarefied practices.

The Taoists feel that it is best for one to begin with the energy of the body, then progress through emotions and thoughts to spiritual power, before going for the ultimate.

B.K. FRANTZIS

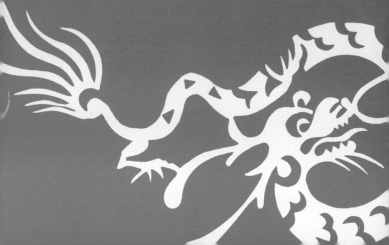

The true essence or root of *chi gong* is, of course, much more than doing forms or breathing exercises. It is an attitude toward life and our own energetic systems. It is an approach toward healthcare and personal lifestyle connecting with the deepest strata of being, down where we all have our origin, the very source of life, sometimes called Tao.

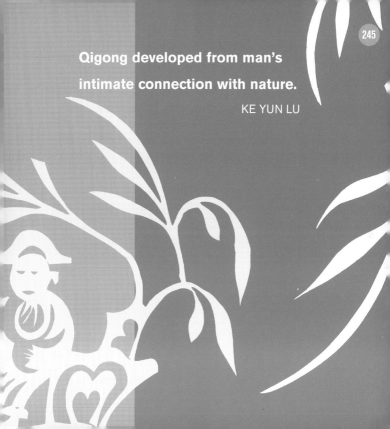

Qigong developed from man's intimate connection with nature.

KE YUN LU

Stand with your back
against the trunk of a tree,
fingers interlaced at the navel.
Now breathe slowly,
from the belly, and try to
open yourself to the living
energy of the tree.
You may be surprised at
how much you feel!

Stand with your feet flat on the earth and, with your mind intent, send down roots from the bottom of your feet, at least three times your height, deep into the earth. In this way you will be able to draw healing energy from the earth up into your body.

Stand or sit facing the sun, eyes closed to protect them. With your mind intent, "inhale" yang energy from the sun down into your lower abdomen three to nine times. Feel this energy heating up your lower *dan tien* and then circulating throughout your body.

Stand or sit facing the moon, with your eyes open or closed and "inhale" the yin energy of the moon into your lower *dan tien* in your abdomen three times. Feel the cool, watery energy of the moon enter you, balancing all the hot centers of your body.

When we do *chi* practices we are linking up with the very source of life. In this way, we can use the power of the greater life force to tone, harmonize, balance, and strengthen our own life force.

How can the universe be alive? Because it is the continual transformation of primal *chi*, the vital energy and living soul of the universe. Primal *chi* functions as the subtle connection of the universe in the same way that the nervous system functions in the human body. It extends itself primordially as the self-nature of the universe.

HUA CHING NI

Chinese thought does not easily distinguish between matter and energy. We might think that Qi is somewhere in between, a kind of matter on the verge of becoming energy, or energy at the point of materializing.

TED J. KAPTCHUCK

Chi is moving in our bodies at all times, keeping us alive. But it can get blocked, just like a dam on a river. When this happens, the result can be pain, low energy, or even tumors. We need to unblock those energy channels so that the *chi* can run smoothly like a mountain stream.

By understanding that all things in the universe are just different expressions of chi, one can see why the sages have always said, "All things are one, and the one is all things." Without the outreach and withdrawal, the giving and returning of chi, the transformation of all things would be impossible.

HUA CHING NI

When our *chi* is low or blocked, we feel depressed or ill and are susceptible to infections, or what the Chinese call "outside evils."

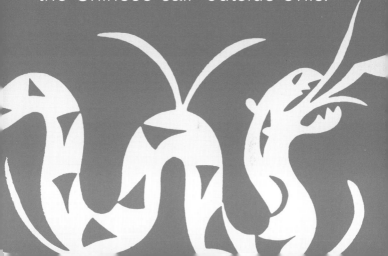

We need to let go of all fear, all attachment, all hope of progress, and all personal theories of spiritual reality and let the *chi* guide us into ever more refined levels of being.

It can take years of practice to heal long-lasting health problems or to build up enough vital *chi* so that new health problems do not occur.

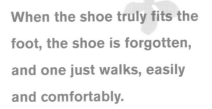

When the shoe truly fits the foot, the shoe is forgotten, and one just walks, easily and comfortably.

B.K. FRANTZIS

The secret to being with the Way or just learning chi movement is to enjoy yourself. The principle of Lao Tzu is "wu wei" which practically speaking means that if you are not too serious about high achievement, you will achieve naturally, just by continuing to practice.

HUA CHING NI

For harmonious attunement, movement is valuable; for careful concentration, stillness is valuable. Movement is patterned on heaven, stillness is patterned on earth; when body and mind are both calm, heaven and earth join.

LI DAOQUN

Real cultivation is only possible in true stillness. In order to refine our energy into more and more subtle levels, we must be able to still the mind, soften the heart, and enter into the deep levels of stillness where true healing can occur.

An easy way to feel *chi* is to create a *chi* ball between your two palms. Hold them out in front of you at shoulder or waist height. Now imagine there is solid ball of energy between them, about the size of a beach ball.

Then gently and slowly bring your hands together, squeezing the ball between them. Next, expand the ball by pulling your hands apart. Do this simple exercise a few times and you will begin to feel a subtle yet solid, rubbery presence between your palms.

A simple yet effective exercise is to stand quietly for a few moments, then bring your arms slowly up in front of you, palms facing down, to shoulder level. Then slowly lower them to waist level. This raises your central *chi* to the heart center, then back down to the lower *dan tien* (field of elixir) center in your lower abdomen. It is an effective way to balance and center your energy. Try it at least nine times and see if you feel a difference in your sense of balance and well-being.

It can take a lifetime of practice to align one's *chi* with the *chi* flow of the universe and to transcend the physical world as we know it, at the point of death or before. But all along the way there are rewards and benefits for anyone who pursues a regular practice.

One of the secrets of a successful *chi gong* practice is that it is frequent and regular. Doing four hours of *chi gong* once a month or even one hour once a week is not as good as doing thirty minutes each day.

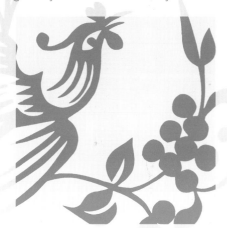

**Many people practicing the Way do it
in the morning then change their minds at night.**

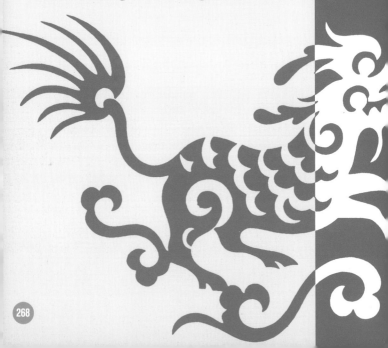

They do it while sitting but then forget it when they stand up, enjoying it momentarily but tiring of it in the long run, starting out diligently but winding up slackening off lazily. Their learning is not clear, their work is not earnest, their hearts are not calm, and their spirits are not true. Although they study for years, they don't attain, and yet they say the Great Way has turned away from humanity.

WANG LIPING

In energy work, learn how to carry the wonderful, calming, and healing energy that we experience when we are doing our practice into the rest of our life—when we are walking the dog, doing the dishes, or sitting at our computer.

Whenever you are doing
energy work, allow
yourself to relax and have
fun with it!

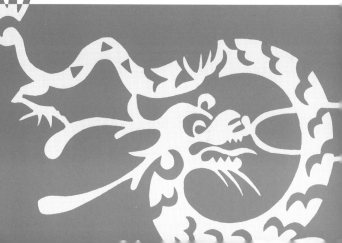

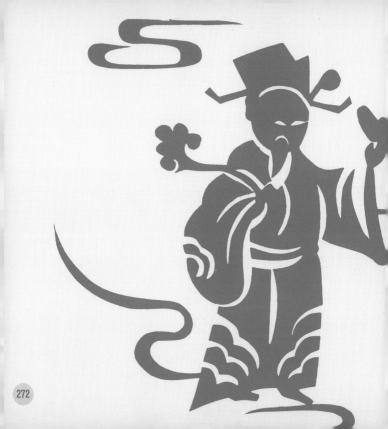

People have different goals. Some people just want a little more energy and a stronger immune system. Others have serious health issues they are dealing with.

A few might wish to go all the way and attain immortality. No matter what your goal is, if you practice sincerely and regularly, your goal can be reached. Even if you don't reach your goal one 100 percent, your life will be changed!

There are many different forms of *chi gong* that can be done moving or standing, in a wheelchair or while lying in a hospital bed. Whatever your situation, there is a practice that is just right for you!

Practicing *chi gong* will make you healthier, emotionally centered, psychologically balanced, more psychic, smarter, more attractive, more creative, and happier; it will strengthen your will and deepen your character.

A powerful medicine that is produced within us, that does not require a doctor's prescription and has no cost, clearly this idea is one of the "health wonders" of the world.

ROGER JAHNKE

Taoist cultivation of *chi* energy may extend into what, at first glance, appears to be impossibly subtle spiritual realms, but it is always with down-to-earth and in-the-body practices.

MANTAK CHIA

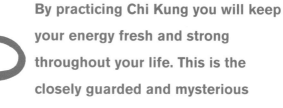

By practicing Chi Kung you will keep your energy fresh and strong throughout your life. This is the closely guarded and mysterious "secret" of Chinese longevity.

JAMES MACRITCHIE

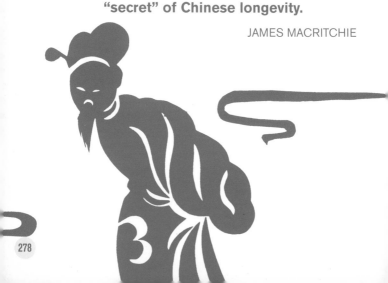

There is an old saying that "*chi* follows *yi*," meaning that *chi* can be directed by the mind. Ancient Taoists knew what modern Western science is only discovering, that we can direct healing energy with our mind and affect the healing process.

The foundation of all *chi gong* practice is the breath. Once we learn how to work with the breath, or, better yet, to begin to allow the breath to do its work unhindered, we can affect great change in our bodies and psyches.

When we practice *chi gong* with the intention of not only healing ourselves but of becoming a healing influence on all those around us, we begin practicing high-level *chi gong*. This enables us to help others become stronger and healthier; they are then freed to help others in an unbroken and endless chain.

If the energy system is operating correctly, if it is balanced and free-flowing with the right quality and good volume, then the emotions will be fully available and appropriate to the particular situation.

If the energy is stuck, blocked, empty, weak, excessive, stagnant, or otherwise out of order in any area, there will be corresponding disturbances and imbalances in the feelings and attitudes.

JIM MACRITCHIE

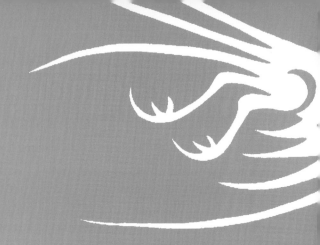

Another form of *chi* or energy work is *tai chi* (*tai ji*), a form of slow-moving dancelike set movements, which has been popular in the West for years. Like other forms of *chi gong*, it works with the principles of rootedness, balance, and the smooth flow of energy throughout the body.

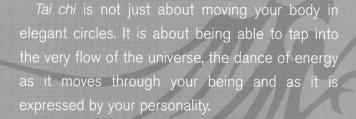

Tai chi is not just about moving your body in elegant circles. It is about being able to tap into the very flow of the universe, the dance of energy as it moves through your being and as it is expressed by your personality.

We can apply the lessons we learn in *tai chi* practice to the rest of our lives, learning when it is best to push forward and when to retreat. Using the principles of emptiness, we can sink or turn at just the right moment so that a blow is met by empty space. This can work emotionally as well as physically.

Eventually, after long years of practice, our energy will become transformed, we will become transformed, and in this way the world will become transformed.

Tai chi helps you find a moving center. It's a movement meditation, you move your center with you. Although you are constantly in motion, you retain that quietness and stillness.

CHUNGLIANG AL HUANG

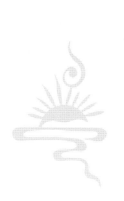

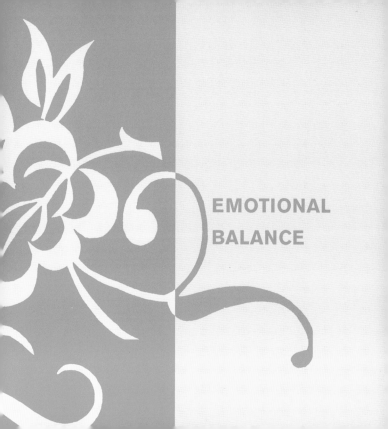

EMOTIONAL
BALANCE

When we speak of emotions on the Path of Tao, we must remember that, to the Taoists, emotions are seen as energy states. And as such, we can learn to have some control over them and thus, over our lives.

By learning how to balance our emotions with meditation, *chi gong*, herbs, acupuncture, and understanding, and by learning to have some objectivity, we become less a victim of our emotions and more the master of them.

Because of this, emotional balance is crucial to our self-cultivation.

We learn to balance our emotions—not by suppressing them or ignoring them—but by learning how to harmonize and transform them. In this way, they become part of our spiritual and energetic practice.

We all have emotions. However spiritual we are, as much as we work on letting go of inappropriate desires, we still have times when we find ourselves falling into a maelstrom of emotion. This is all natural. It is in how we deal with these emotions and just how large a part they play in our lives that makes the difference.

The difficulty of being spiritual is not because you are not moral enough, or you are not spiritual enough, but because you are captive to your emotions.

HUA CHING NI

Worrying about the future
will only cause distress in the
present. Despairing about
the past will only cripple you in
the present. By living primarily
in the eternal now, you can have
power over both the past
and the future.

There is nothing worse than not
knowing when one has enough.
There is no greater fault than
the desire for things.
The one who knows when
enough is enough will always
have enough.

LAO TZU

It is important to remember that emotions are energy states. Thus they can either contribute to our energy or deplete it. By not attempting to harmonize our emotions we do ourselves a great energetic disservice.

By not investing too much energy into any one specific emotional state, positive or negative, we can become free of the energetic influences of that state. We can then learn how to become masters of our emotions rather than slaves to them.

It is when we allow ourselves to go to extremes with our emotions that we lose control. Better to find the middle place, neither extreme joy nor extreme sorrow, so that we can dwell in peace.

In the great tradition of Tao,
you are asked to maintain
your childlike heart.

HUA CHING NI

Be simple, be open,
don't be afraid to be silly,
don't be afraid to be wrong,
don't be afraid to be judged,
don't be afraid to be foolish,
and you will gain the
wisdom of Tao.

The baby looks at things all day without squinting and staring; that is because his eyes are not focused on any particular object. He goes without knowing where he is going, and stops without knowing what he is doing. He merges himself with the surroundings and goes along with them. These are the principles of mental hygiene.

CHUANG TZU

Those who know do not speak.

Those who speak do not know.

LAO TZU

There is a difference between childlike and childish. The follower of the Path of Tao is still in touch with the wonder, the magic and the excitement of the childlike state. They are open to new experiences, new ideas, and new adventures. On the other hand, they are not petty, selfish, self-absorbed, or prone to throwing fits of rage when they don't get their way.

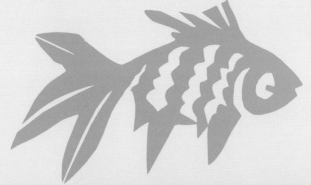

By not allowing ourselves
the luxury of having
opinions about everything
we can free up our
emotional selves to deal
simply with what is.

Wise people are generally those who speak little. They don't feel the need to boast about their accomplishments. They don't need to put on great emotional displays but rather conduct themselves in a quiet, humble manner.

By simplifying, by surrendering to the moment, by putting aside past prejudices, and by allowing our heart to soften we are better able to see into the emotional core of our life and allow all our actions to come from a sense of balance and harmony.

If practitioners of the Tao can look upon the life of essence as the one important thing, see through material objects and cut through attachments at one stroke, then all things will be empty to them and they will be free. Not obsessed with food and clothing, not in a turmoil over worldly affairs, letting all vexations and problems run their natural course, leaving life and death up to fate, acting with nobility, maintaining an iron will, with this firmness one can finish what one begins; growing stronger with time, one has direction and purpose.

LIU I-MING

It is not easy to be masters of our emotions. But if we are not, our lives will be run by them and we will always be victims of our own unhealthy emotional states.

We need to find a way to be objective about our emotions. By approaching them as energy states we can more easily regulate them. Then we can use them creatively instead of being slaves to them.

A bad emotional habit many of us have is leaning too heavily on others for our own emotional well-being. If we are too easily influenced by others we will never have the emotional independence it takes for serious self-cultivation.

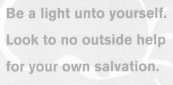

Be a light unto yourself.
Look to no outside help
for your own salvation.

THE BUDDHA

Taoists are not "followers." They do not spend their time searching for leaders or gurus. Instead they take the time to look within to find their own answers.

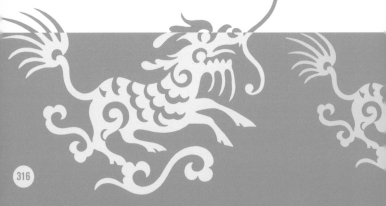

Saving the world starts

with saving yourself.

HUA CHING NI

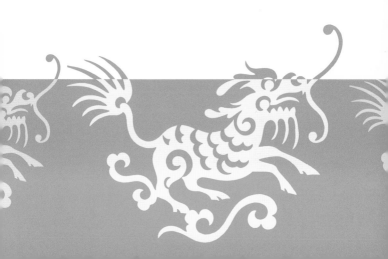

If you are not emotionally
healthy yourself, how can
you hope to be of service
to anyone else?

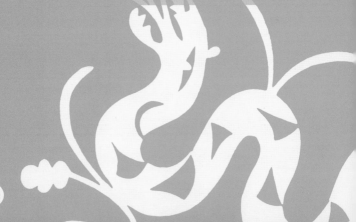

Once there was a man who lost his axe and was sure that the boy who lived next door had stolen it. By observing the boy's actions very carefully over several days the man convinced himself that the boy had the look of a thief.

Then, while walking through the forest, the man found his axe. When he returned home and again saw the boy next door he suddenly realized that the boy did not look like a thief after all.

LIEH TZU

When you start to feel yourself "losing it" emotionally, stop, breathe slowly, from the belly. Remember that this moment will pass.

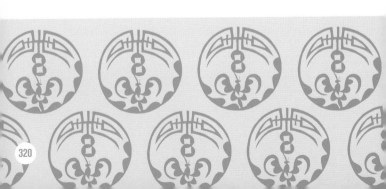

It is when we lose our objectivity that our emotions carry us away. What on one day can seem like a small problem, on another can seem like an insurmountable challenge.

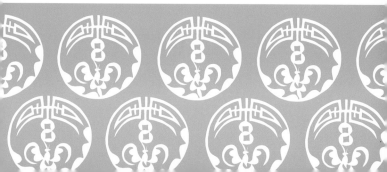

Whatever may have happened to you in the past can be changed or at least altered by your actions in the present.

A Taoist conserves his energy easily
by according with and adapting
himself to each situation.

HUA CHING NI

Remember, an emotional response or action that is appropriate for one situation may not be appropriate for another. An emotional response or action that is appropriate for one day may not even be appropriate for another.

It is the Taoist's ability to live wholly or as much as possible in the present that is his or her greatest strength.

When we are born we are weak and tender.

When we die we are hard and stiff.

Green plants are soft and fragile.

At their death they are dry and brittle.

Therefore the hard and stiff are the
followers of death.

The soft and weak are the followers of life.

LAO TZU

The secret of the emotional "martial artist" is that, when she is greeted with force, she responds with softness. In this way, the force has no way to keep going and will run out on its own.

What is flexibility? If someone strikes you, you endure it meekly; if someone reviles you, you greet it with a smile. Unconcerned by illness, not entering into judgments, being courteous and humble, getting rid of arrogance, gradually dispelling force of habit, noticing your own faults at all times, checking your own state in all situations, being careful about what you have not perceived, acting in accord with your basic state and not wishing for anything else, you are not concerned with human sentiments or worldly affairs, you sweep away all false thoughts and idle imaginations, leaving not a trace.

LIU I-MING

The present is the point of power. It is far more powerful than anything in the past or the future. If we can free ourselves from the constraints of our past or worries about the future and focus on the present, we will make informed, intelligent decisions about our life.

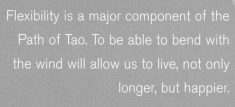

Flexibility is a major component of the
Path of Tao. To be able to bend with
the wind will allow us to live, not only
longer, but happier.

As nothing is permanent, there is nothing to take seriously. As there is nothing to take seriously, we should laugh at the world. As we laugh at the world, we should realize that understanding the changing nature of life is the swiftest way to joy.

DENG MING DAO

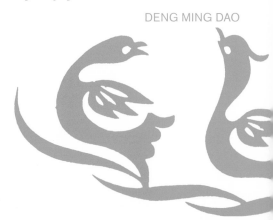

When we can learn to laugh
at the world with all its
endless distractions and
disasters, we can better
learn to laugh at ourselves,
a sure sign of enlightenment.

I like to believe that, for as long as the world contains wonderers and wanderers who are frugal in their habits, lovers of people in their endless vitality, sincere in their pursuit of truth and able to laugh at themselves, the spirit of Taoism will live on.

JOHN BLOFELD

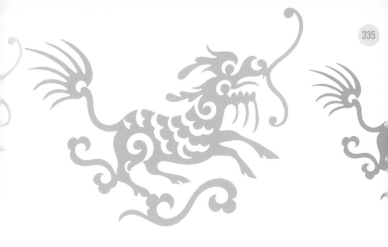

By allowing ourselves to go with
the flow of each unfolding moment
we will not be as easily knocked
off course when we hit the rapids.

The student asked the teacher, "I am poor, I have not eaten meat nor drunk wine for many months. Can this be considered fasting?"

"That," answered his teacher, "is only the fasting that one does for sacrificial ceremonies. It is not the fasting of the mind."

"What is this fasting of the mind?" asked the student.

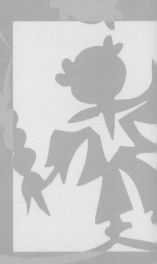

"In fasting of the mind your will must become strong. You do not listen with your ears but with your mind. You do not only listen with your mind but with your vital energy. Your ears can only hear, your mind can only think, but your vital energy is empty and receptive to all things. Since the Tao abides in emptiness, you will then reach the Tao. This is fasting of the mind."

CHUANG TZU

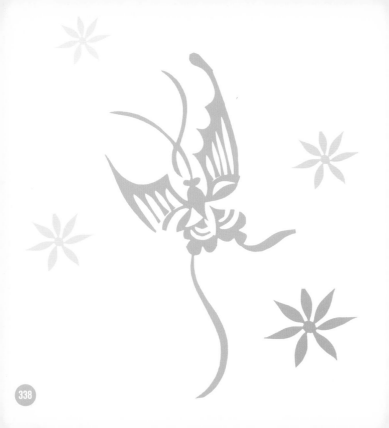

When we learn to listen, not with our ears, but with our heart or our *chi*, we can better discern the proper response. When we get our judgmental mind out of the way, we can respond fully, from our own essential nature.

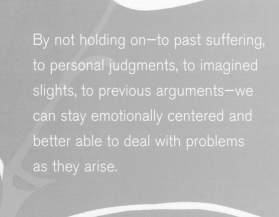

By not holding on—to past suffering, to personal judgments, to imagined slights, to previous arguments—we can stay emotionally centered and better able to deal with problems as they arise.

A sorrow shared
is a sorrow halved.
A joy shared is a
joy doubled.

Remember *wu wei*, the art of doing without doing. By accepting every experience that comes our way, without judgment, and without putting a positive or negative value on it, we can be fully in the moment and at peace with ourselves and the world.

Not to have feeling is inhuman.

To be carried away by feeling is foolish.

Not to have desire is death.

To be a slave to desire is to be lost.

DENG MING DAO

By accepting what
we cannot change,
by changing what we
can, and by learning to
discern the difference,
we can take control of
our emotional life.

Unlike Indian philosophies, neither of the great Chinese philosophies, Confucianism and Taoism, can be called pessimistic; both assume, not that life is misery, but that joy and misery alternate like day and night, each having its proper place in the world order.

A.C. GRAHAM

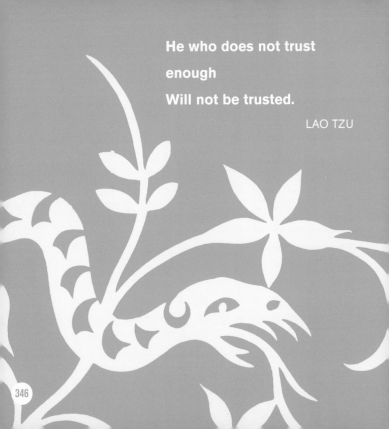

He who does not trust
enough
Will not be trusted.

LAO TZU

To be able to trust in what
we cannot see,
to be able to believe in what
we cannot understand,
to be able to practice what
we do not yet know—
in this way are we able to
choose this and not that.

Chuang Tzu and Hui Tzu were crossing the Hao river when Chuang Tzu said to his friend, "These fish we see below us come out and swim about so leisurely. This is the joy of fishes."

His friend turned to him and said, "How do you know what fish enjoy, you're not a fish?"

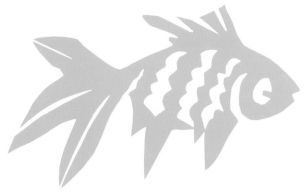

"You are not me," answered Chuang Tzu, "so how do you know what I know about the joy of fish?"

"Well," said his friend, somewhat indignantly. "I am not you and so do not know what you know. But, as you are certainly not a fish, there is no possible way that you can know what fish enjoy."

"Ah then," said Chuang Tzu. "Let us go back to the beginning of our conversation. When you asked me 'How can you know what fish enjoy' you knew that I did know. The reason I know this is by walking over the river!"

CHUANG TZU

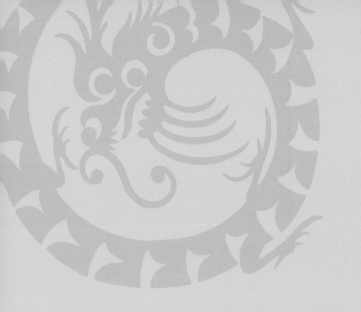

The secret of sagehood, which is
also immortality, is acceptance.

JOHN BLOFELD

We can always learn
much more by merely
observing than by asking
too many questions.

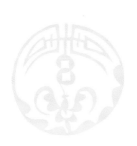

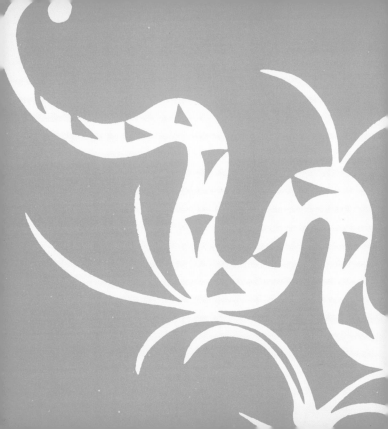

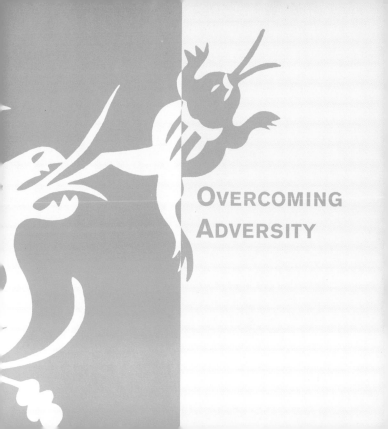

OVERCOMING ADVERSITY

Life is full of challenges, and it is how we rise to each occasion that marks our character. Unfortunately, the old saying that suffering builds character is true. Perhaps it is only in suffering or in being challenged that we are forced to grow and expand our sense of ourselves and, in this way, build the character we need to become sages.

We should look at our suffering as tools for growth, as medicine for our own unhealthy minds, as impetus for change.

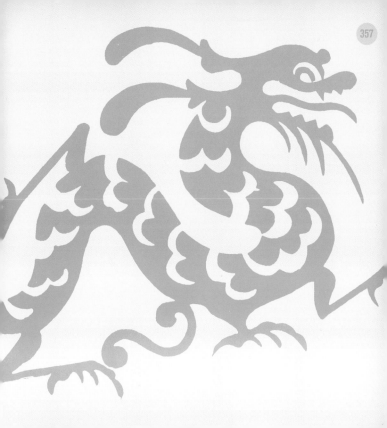

We can use our suffering as the "kick in the butt" that we need to get ourselves out of our daily rut, and then we can learn how to treasure it.

Life is full of suffering. But if we learn how to blend our sufferings and our joys we can then come to an understanding of life. If we don't become too disturbed by our downs or too carried away by our highs we can learn how to find a sort of emotional middle ground. Perhaps then we can learn to dwell in the midst of some kind of serenity.

Adversity is always with us, no matter what station in life we are born into. We have no control over the world around us. Though we may be cocreators of our own lives, much that we end up experiencing seems to be arbitrary and even chaotic.

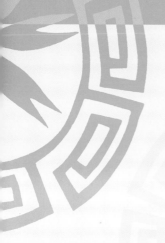

But, while we may have no control over what comes our way, we do have some small control over our responses to it. This, in the end, is our only power, but it is a great power indeed.

While the difference between favor

and disgrace

May seem frightening,

Learn to accept suffering as a part of life.

The reason we suffer

Is because we have a body.

If we didn't have a body,

We would not suffer.

Those who honor their own life

As much as the world itself,

Can be entrusted with the world.

LAO TZU

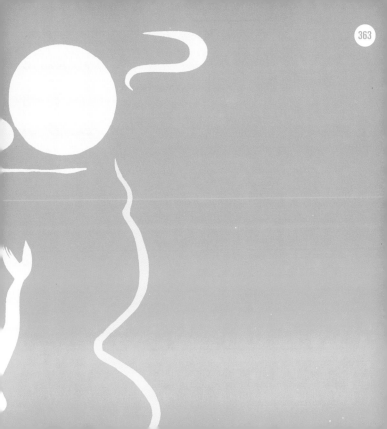

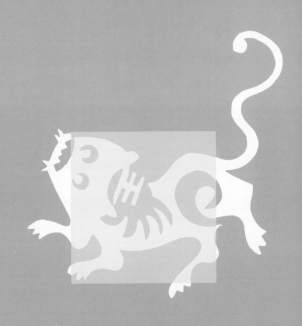

Suffering accompanies life, but love is affirmation.

DENG MING DAO

For those who have no sense of the divine, no connection to the eternal, life is full of danger and suffering. When tragedy strikes, they have no way to cope, they have nothing to fall back upon.

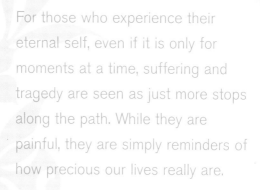

For those who experience their eternal self, even if it is only for moments at a time, suffering and tragedy are seen as just more stops along the path. While they are painful, they are simply reminders of how precious our lives really are.

That most of us experience a
sense of loneliness, of apartness
both from the highest reality and
from all the beings and objects
around us, is due to deluded
understanding and a faulty
sense of perception.

JOHN BLOFELD

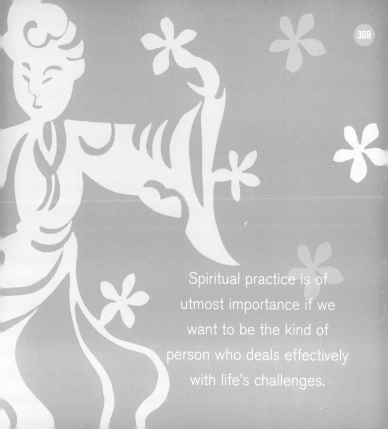

Spiritual practice is of utmost importance if we want to be the kind of person who deals effectively with life's challenges.

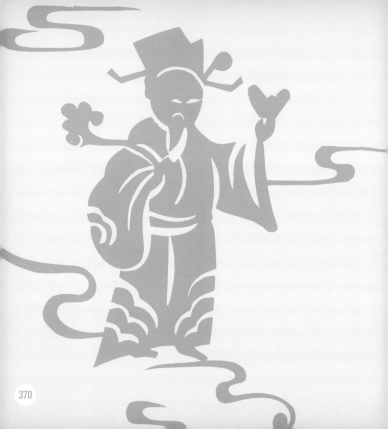

The master had preached for many years that life was but an illusion. Then, when his son died, he wept. His students came to him and said, "Master, how can you weep so when you have told us so many times that all things in this life are illusion?"

"Yes," said the Master, wiping away his tears while they continued to course down his ancient cheeks, "but he was such a beautiful illusion!"

To the Taoist, everything is holy, sacred, miraculous! To the followers of the Way there is no difference between the sacred and the profane.

The highest achievement as a Taoist is the refinement of one's spirit into an irresistible precious sword which can cut through all mental obstacles and impediments.

HUA CHING NI

Many of our so-called problems originate in our minds. It is our worries about the future, our dwelling on past injustices, our constant analyzing of every facet of our lives that creates much of our suffering.

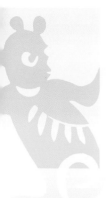

By practicing meditation, by stilling the mind, by allowing ourselves a break once in a while from the wildly leaping "monkey mind," we can experience some sense of peacefulness.

It is not that spiritual people have no problems. They just don't see their problems as necessarily problematical!

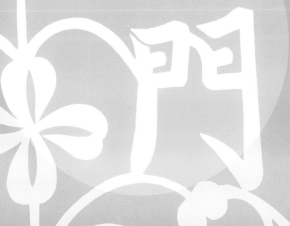

Man should bring the spiritual down to earth and raise the earth to the spiritual.

J.C. COOPER

Eternal truth is very simple and very clear and does not come with any emotional or psychological baggage or attachments.

The world's problem is that
people have become
disconnected from their own
spiritual energy.

HUA CHING NI

As Taoists we are artists of life. We are creators of our own masterpieces, directors of our own movies, writers of our own stories. We all want to be loved and to love. We all want to be happy and to be able to give happiness to others. We all want to be safe, to be whole, to be healthy.

When people lose

their sense of awe,

Disaster follows.

LAO TZU

Best be still, best be empty.
In stillness and emptiness, we find
where to abide;
Taking and giving, we lose the place.

LIEH TZU

When negative experiences come your way it's best if you can deal with them as they are. In other words, don't give them any more power over you than they already have. Stop, or at least slow down, deal with them, then move on.

The teaching of spiritual alchemy says that when the mind runs off one should gather it in; having gathered it in, then let go of it. After action, seek rest; finding rest, one develops enlightenment. Who says that one cannot find tranquility in the midst of clamor and activity?

CHANG SAN FENG

In the old days spiritual seekers went off into the mountains to escape the "world of dust." Today it is important that we learn to do our spiritual and emotional cultivation in the midst of the world. In this way we can have some affect on those around us as well.

There was once a very rich man who had many servants, whom he worked from dawn to dusk. One of his servants was an old man who, each night, dreamed that he was a rich man, living a life of leisure. Then, upon waking, he would feel refreshed and happy and thus could work all day without getting tired.

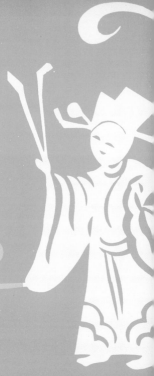

Meanwhile, the rich man went to sleep each night and dreamed that he was a lowly servant, breaking his back all day long under the hot sun. He would toss and turn, sweat and groan all night long and woke up each morning more tired than the night before.

When he complained to his friends they told him, "Don't worry. By night you may suffer but by day you are a rich man, well respected in the business community, and you have far more than you will ever need. You are at the top of the ladder; that is why you dream at night that you are at the bottom. You cannot have it both ways. Things must balance. That is why you have those vexing dreams."

After thinking about this the rich man decided to give his servants more time off and a lighter load. After this, he began to sleep more soundly and his nightmares went away.

LIEH TZU

The answers to all our questions are hidden everywhere, just outside our line of sight—that is, until we open our eyes a little wider and begin looking around us instead of just straight ahead. Then they jump out at us from everywhere, displaying themselves in all their stunning simplicity.

The wise one dwells on the deep meaning
And not the flashy surface.
They prefer the fruit over the flower.

LAO TZU

By discerning the real meaning in each action or situation the follower of the Tao is able to ignore the obvious and instead dwell on what is eternal.

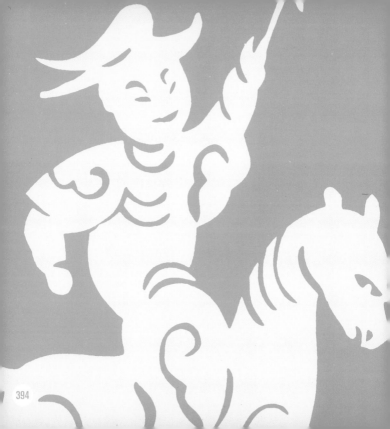

Those who understand others have wisdom,
Those who understand themselves have enlightenment.
Those who master others have power,
Those who master themselves have inner strength.

LAO TZU

We must delve deeply into our own natures before we can presume to understand others. We must learn how to master our own emotional states before we can correctly interpret others.

Suffering is inevitable. We all suffer. It is in how we suffer that sets the sage apart from the ordinary person. It is when we employ "creative suffering" that we can utilize our suffering for our own greater good.

When conflict comes
our way we are given
the opportunity to bring
forth aspects of our
own personality that
may usually lie dormant.
It is a chance to see
ourselves in a new light.

Those who are intent on finding disagreement will usually find it. While those who go out of their way to find a place of agreement, find that they have many friends and few enemies.

It is by applying the principles of yin and yang that we can be more effective in dealing with adversity. According to yin and yang, there is a time for moving aggressively forward just as there is a time to be more yin and hold back. No one approach works every time. Each situation must be considered in its own light.

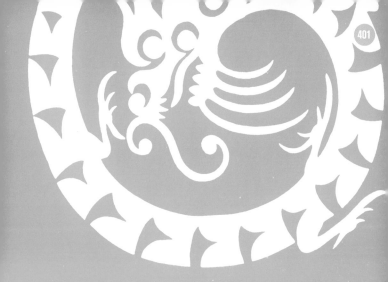

Then again, sometimes the best thing
to do is to do nothing! It is much like a
stream of water that runs up against a
dam. There the current is stopped.

The water can't go any further until the level rises up over the top of the dam.

This is the situation where we feel stuck, where nothing seems to be happening for us. We may be tempted to try and force something to happen. But that can often cause disaster.

Instead of flinging ourselves against the rocks, we must simply sit and wait. Even though we may feel that nothing is changing, in reality it is. If we wait long enough, and patiently enough our energy levels will rise and we will be able to move forward again with new strength and vigor.

If the force of the other is too great, then deflect it, but do not surrender your intention and do not let go. Come back, just as the bamboo comes back after it has been pressed by the wind. If your opponent pushes you far, be prepared to go just a little further still, so that your opponent is exhausted. Then reassert yourself in the correct measure.

DENG MING DAO

We who follow Tao
make use of whatever
comes our way–and that
includes conflict.

DENG MING DAO

If someone comes at you with an aggressive yang force, simply deflect it with the opposite yin force. For example, if someone begins an argument with you, you can choose to respond in a yang way and keep up the argument or you can respond in a yin fashion and either find the point of agreement or just refuse to keep up your end of the argument. Remember, it takes two to argue!

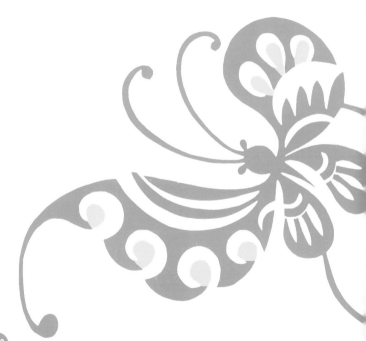

If you want to be a leader of people,
Conduct yourself as though you are
below them.
If you want to lead them forward,
Do so from behind.
In this way people will not find you
oppressive.
You can stand before them
And they will not be harmed.
In this way everyone will be glad to
support you.
By not contending,
You will not be contended with.

LAO TZU

If one understands the concept of yin and yang, how can there be yielding without assertion? One cannot be yielding forever.

DENG MING DAO

It is only through long and deep self study that we can learn our strengths and weaknesses so that we are better able to respond appropriately to each situation.

The frequency radiating from one's own mind and spirit creates an attraction for the universal energies of the corresponding frequencies, which invariably echo back as the ingredients of one's own daily experience.

HUA CHING NI

When we plant seeds of discord, we will see the fruits of discord. When we plant the seeds of peace, peace will enter our lives.

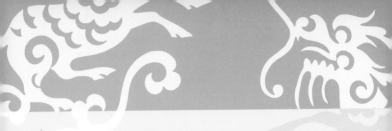

Achieve success, but without vanity.

Achieve success, but without aggression.

Achieve success, but without arrogance.

Achieve success, but without gain;

Achieve success, but without force.

You may feel strong now,

But in time you will become old and weak.

That which goes against the Tao

Will come to an early end.

LAO TZU

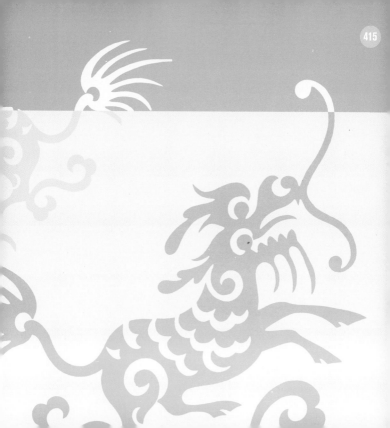

Life is full of obstacles and adversity. Some of it is self-created, some of it just a part of life. Remember, it is how we respond to difficulties that determines our spiritual character.

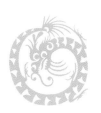

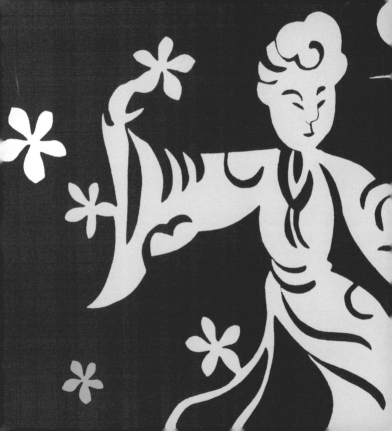

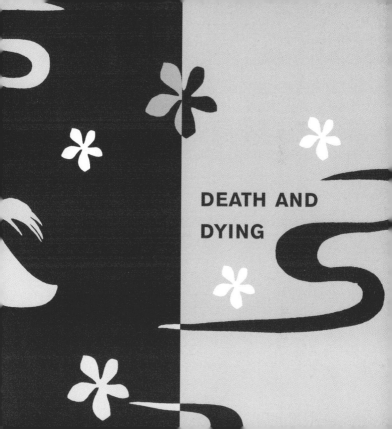

DEATH AND
DYING

Taoists do not see death as an end but as another beginning, much as each year brings the seasons, which die into the next only to be reborn again. The ancient Taoist masters were men and women who gained their knowledge from observing the world of Nature.

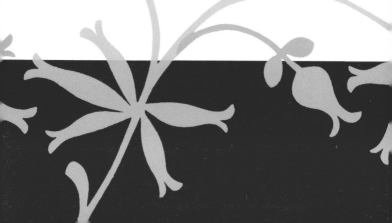

They paid close attention to the cycles of the seasons, the round of birth, death, and rebirth that comes with each passing year. They watched as the new seedlings, from deep within the dark earth, sprouted forth into the light, only to die again at the end of each season.

They recognized their own lives as a part of this pattern. They saw that all of life is involved in birth, death, and rebirth.

From their deep meditations the Taoist masters were able to discern different spirits that resided within us. They called them *hun* and *po*.

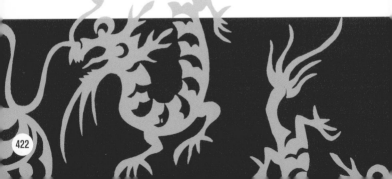

At the point of death some spirits went back into the earth, the source of our own lives. The rest ascended into the spiritual realm. Whatever spiritual cultivation each person had reached caused the spiritual souls to be reconnected with the life force and become incarnated again.

People who learn Tao recognize that the next part of their lives, each new coming decade, and even each next moment is a newly reincarnated life.

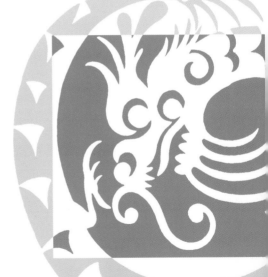

If time is actually circular, as is described in most mystical texts, and not linear, then we are living all our past, present, and future lives simultaneously. Those glimpses into the past or future that we sometimes are rewarded with are merely connection points between levels.

The past isn't different from today, because we know what began in the past. And today isn't different from the past, because we know where today came from. What is neither being nor comes from anywhere else we call the thread that has no end. This is the thread of the Tao.

LU HUI-CHING

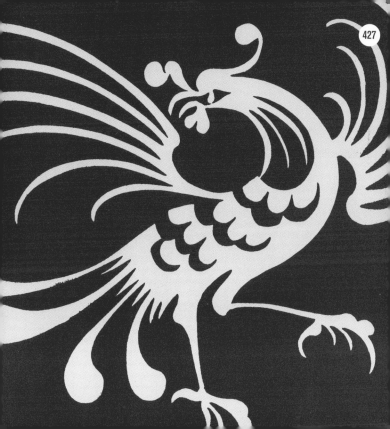

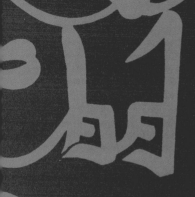

**To be born normally,
coming from nowhere,
is the Way.**

LIEH TZU

**To die normally, in accordance with
your manner of life, is also the Way.**

LIEH TZU

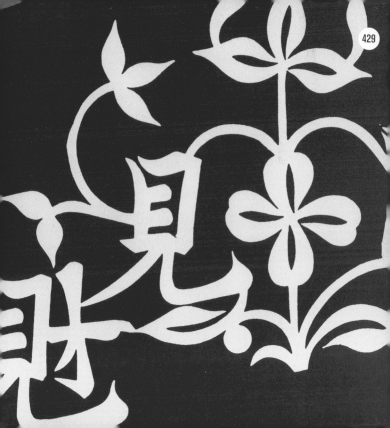

We fear death as we fear the unknown. It is why we fear the dark.

Dying is the virtue in us going to its destination.

LIEH TZU

It is by being eternally present
that we are able to transcend
what we think of as time.
And in that experience of each
eternally present moment,
death does not exist.

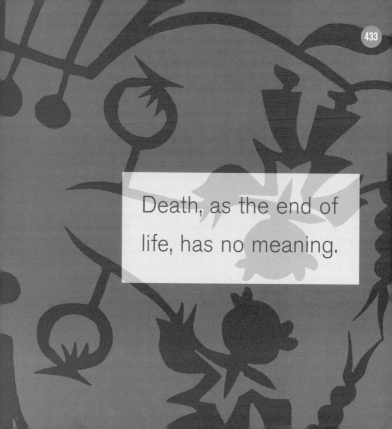

Death, as the end of life, has no meaning.

Upon hearing of the death of Chuang Tzu's wife, his good friend Hui Tzu went over to comfort him and found the sage sitting on the ground banging on an overturned pot and singing a song at the top of his lungs.

Horrified at such behavior, Hui Tzu reproved him, saying, "This woman has lived with you, borne your children, grown old with you, and now she has died. It is bad enough not to be weeping at this time but to be out here banging on a pot and singing is too much!"

Chuang Tzu replied, "You are mistaken my friend, at first I could not help but feel sad and depressed at my beloved wife's death. But then I began to reflect. In the beginning, she had no life, and having no life she had no spirit, and having no spirit she had no body.

But then she was given life, she was given a spirit and then she was given a body. Now things have changed again and she is dead. She has joined the great cycle of the seasons, from spring to autumn to winter to summer.

Now she lies suspended between heaven and earth. Why then should I weep and moan over her. It would be as though I did not understand the process of life. Therefore I stopped and decided to celebrate."

CHUANG TZU

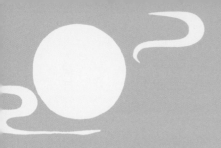

How do I know that in clinging to this life I'm not merely clinging to a dream and delaying my entry into the real world?

CHUANG TZU

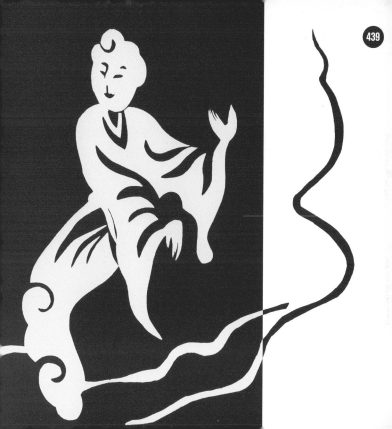

The great earth burdens me
with a body, causes me to toil
in life, eases me in old age,
and rests me in death. That
which makes my life good,
makes my death good.

CHUANG TZU

Taoists are always, and in all ways, concerned with doing things in the proper order, in the proper timing, in the proper manner. From birth to death, if we pay attention to the timing, we may perhaps become masters over time ourselves and live as immortals.

There is a certain quality of illusion in this world of ours. The ancients called it "the play of the gods," viewing life as some sort of cosmic joke. If this is so, we can look at death as the ultimate punch line!

When one dies, one knows the right time to go and is prepared to make the transition, and there is no life separate from the deep, eternal Tao.

HUA CHING NI

When the Master died, Chin Shih came to the funeral, looked around and shouted three times.

One of the other disciples said, "I thought you were a friend of the Master."

"Yes, of course I am," replied Chin Shih.

"Well, do you think it proper to behave this way?" asked the disciple.

"Yes," said Chin Shih. "When I first walked into the room I thought that the Master's spirit was still here. Now I see that it is not. I came prepared to mourn but, upon seeing everyone here wailing at the top of their lungs, I realized that this was all wrong. This is ignoring the natural course of things.

The Master came because it was his time. When it was his time to leave, he left. If we ourselves are also content to follow the natural flow there would be no room for grief. This is truly freedom from bondage. When the wood burns the wood itself is consumed, to where it goes we cannot say."

CHUANG TZU

The ancient sages knew that life was eternal and that death was not an end but just the beginning of a new cycle. Therefore they did not rejoice at birth or wail at death.

They saw both birth and death as part of the cycle of things. They had no fear of death but saw it only as a new beginning, an opportunity to return to the spiritual world, a way to be "recycled" back into the Tao.

Life consists of cycles within cycles. One day we're up, the next day we're down. If we don't try to hold on too tightly, we will not suffer as much.

Taoists believe that when we die, we then merge again with the origin of all life. Our personality is "recycled" back into Tao. But our energy, especially our spiritual energy, that we have built through self-cultivation lives on, to be reborn into another life, until we have attained immortality.

Often the way we live fashions the way that we die. If we learn to surrender to each unfolding moment in life we will be better able to surrender to the great transformation of death.

Tzu Lao lay dying, surrounded by his wife and children, who were all weeping. His friend Tzu Li came to see him, and, finding them thus, said to his family, "Be quiet, do not disturb him in his time of great transformation!" Then he spoke to his friend saying, "Great is the creator of life. What will he make you in your next life do you think, the liver of a rat, or a bug's leg?" Tzu Lao smiled and answered, "The relationship of a child to his parents is that he follows their directions, no matter where they lead. The relationship of yin and yang are even more important than that. If they urge me to die now, I must humbly submit, otherwise I am being obstinate and rebellious. The great earth gives me a form, I toil on it, in my old age I find my ease on it, and at death I am able to rest in it. That which makes my life good also makes my death good."

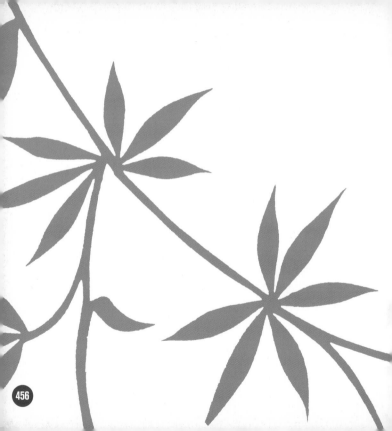

In reality, it is not that the
Great Way turns away
from anyone; but people
themselves turn their
own backs on the Way.

WANG LIPING

It is said that we are born
from a quiet sleep and that
at death, we slip into a calm
awakening.

CHUANG TZU

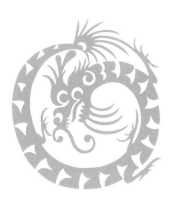

Bibliography

Beinfield, Harriet, and Efrem Korngold. *Between Heaven and Earth: A Guide to Chinese Medicine.* New York: Ballentine Books, 1991.

Blofeld, John. *The Secret and Sublime: Taoist Mysteries and Magic.* New York: Dutton, 1973.

Chia, Mantak and Maneewan. *Fusion of the Five Elements.* Huntington, N.Y.: Healing Tao Books, 1989.

Chia, Mantak. *Taoist Ways to Transform Stress into Vitality.* Huntington, N.Y.: Healing Tao Books, 1985.

Chu, Wen Kuan, trans. *Tao and Longevity: Mind-Body Transformation.* York Beach, Mass.: Samuel Weiser, Inc.,1984

Connelly, Dianne M. *All Sickness Is Home Sickness.* Columbia, Md.: Centre for Traditional Acupuncture, 1986.

Feng, Gia-Fu and Jane English, trans. *Chuang Tsu: Inner Chapters.* New York: Vintage, 1974.

Feng, Gia-Fu and Jane English, trans. *Lao Tsu: Tao Te Ching.* New York: Alfred A. Knopf, 1972.

Frantzis, B. K. *Opening The Energy Gates of Your Body: Gain Lifelong Vitality.* Berkeley, Calif.: North Atlantic Books, 1993.

Garripoli, Garri. *Qigong: Essence of the Healing Dance*. Deerfeild Park, Fla.: Health Communications, Inc., 1999.

Kaptchuk, Ted J. *The Web That Has No Weaver: Understanding Chinese Medicine*. Chicago: Contemporary Books, 2000.

Kohn, Livia. *The Taoist Experience: An Anthology*. New York: State University of New York Press, 1993.

MacRitchie, James. *Chi Kung: Cultivating Personal Energy*. Rockport, Mass: Element Books, 1993.

Ni, Hua-Ching. *8,000 Years of Wisdom: Conversations with Taoist Master Ni, Hua Ching, Book I*. Los Angeles: The Shrine of the Eternal Breath of Tao and College of Tao and Traditional Chinese Healing, 1983.

Ni, Hua-Ching. *8,000 Years of Wisdom: Conversations with Taoist Master Ni, Hua Ching, Book III*. Los Angeles: The Shrine of the Eternal Breath of Tao and College of Tao and Traditional Chinese Healing, 1983.

Ni, Hua-Ching. *Moonlight In The Dark Night*. Los Angeles: The Shrine of the Eternal Breath of Tao and College of Tao and Traditional Chinese Healing, 1991.

Ni, Hua-Ching. *Power of Natural Healing*. Los Angeles: The Shrine of the Eternal Breath of Tao and College of Tao and Traditional Chinese Healing, 1990.

Ni, Hua-Ching. *The Taoist Inner View of the Universe and the Immortal Realm*. Los Angeles: The Shrine of the Eternal Breath of Tao and College of Tao and Traditional Chinese Healing, 1979.

Ni, Maoshing. *The Yellow Emperor's Classic of Medicine*. Boston: Shambala, 1995.

Olson, Stuart Alve, trans. *The Jade Emperor's Mind Seal Classic*. St. Paul, Minn.: Dragon Door, 1992.

Palmer, Martin. *The Elements of Taoism*. Rockport, Mass.: Element, 1991.

Reid, Daniel. *The Complete Guide to Chi-Kung*. Boston: Shambhala, 1998.

Reid, Daniel. *The Shambala Guide to Traditional Chinese Medicine*. Boston: Shambhala, 1996.

Yu-Lan, Fung. *A Short History of Chinese Philosophy*. New York: Macmillan, 1948.

Solala Towler is a musican, poet, and teacher. He is editor of *The Empty Vessel, A Journal of Contemporary Taoism*, a magazine with an international subscription and distribution base (www.abodetao.com). He is also author of *A Gathering of Cranes: Bringing the Tao to the West and Embarking On the Way: A Guide to Western Taoism*. He is an instructor of Taoist meditation and of several styles of *chi gong*. He has taught classes and seminars all over the U.S. and abroad and is currently President of the National Qigong Association o USA.

Solala leads yearly tours to China to study *chi gong*, and visit Taoist temples and sacred mountains. You can email him at solala@abodetao.com or call (001)-541-345-8854.

First published by MQ Publications Limited
12 The Ivories, 6–8 Northhampton St., London, N1 2HY

Copyright © MQ Publications Limited 2002
Text © Solala Towler 2002
Design: Axis Design Editions

All materials quoted from the works of Hua Ching Ni are reprinted, with
permission, by SevenStar Communications., 13315 W. Washington Blvd.,
Ste. 200, Los Angeles, CA 90066

Library of Congress Cataloging-in-Publication Data
Towler, Solala
    Tao paths to long life/Solala Towler
        p.cm.
    ISBN: 0–7407–2294–8
    1. Eternity. 2. Tao. I. Title.

BT912.T68 2002
299.5144–dc21   2001046434

Printed and bound in China